HAPPY PEOPLE RARELY GET CANCER

by

J. I. Rodale

RODALE PRESS, INC.

Emmaus, Penna. 18049

STANDARD BOOK NUMBER 87596-047-2

LIBRARY OF CONGRESS CATALOG CARD NUMBER 78-127177

PRINTED IN THE UNITED STATES

G-470

FIRST PRINTING—OCTOBER, 1970

Table of Contents

Chapter		Page
1.	Sir Heneage Ogilvie	1
2.	Gardeners and Cancer	8
3.	The Happy Hunzas	13
4.	The Nagyri	21
5.	Roseto, Pennsylvania	29
6.	Emotions May Have Cancer Link	42
7.	Blood Sugar Affects Your Emotions	48
8.	Personality and the Thyroid	59
9.	Pinning Down the Cancer Personality	68
10.	Are Suicide and Cancer Related?	77
11.	Dr. Gotthard Booth's Writings	83
12.	Dr. Elida Evans	89
13.	Some Comments by Doctors	121
14.	A Recent Study	129
15.	Isolation and Hodgkin's Disease	137
16.	Repression and Lung Cancer	148
17.	Personal Loss and the Lymphatics	158
18.	Mothers, Daughters and Leukemia	165
19.	Nuns Live Longer	170
20.	The Exaltation of Walking	177
21.	A Healthy Mind in a Healthy Body	187
22.	Raising Happier Children	195
23.	Conclusion	202

CHAPTER 1

Sir Heneage Ogilvie

IN LATE 1959 I was reading a new book entitled *No Miracles Among Friends,* published by Maxfield Parrish of London, and written by Sir Heneage Ogilvie, a famous British surgeon. It had something in it that made me sit up and take notice. It was that the happy man never gets cancer. Here is how Sir Heneage puts it:

"The happy man never gets cancer. I have often caught myself thinking about a colleague. 'So and so has started to look unhappy. He is either unhappy because he has got cancer, or he is going to get cancer because he is unhappy.' So run my thoughts, and I try to dismiss them. Then I notice that he is missing from the next council meeting. Three months later I read his obituary in *The British Medical Journal.*"

This was very interesting to me because up to this time I had considered only nutrition and exercise as factors in producing good health. Now here was a conservative member of a conservative profession of a conservative country saying that the mind or the spirit was also a possible cause of good health.

Dr. Ogilvie went on: "The instances where the first recognizable onset of cancer has followed almost immediately on some disaster, a bereavement, the break-up of a relationship, a financial crisis, or an accident, are so numerous that they suggest that some controlling force that has hitherto kept this outbreak of cell communism in check has been removed. The late appearance of secondaries, suggesting that over the years some undetected cancer cells have been lying latent and kept in check by some unknown restraining force, is commonplace after operations for cancer of the breast. Very often, indeed, so often as to suggest that if the true cause could be discovered, the treatment of cancer might be unravelled, the signal for renewed growth seems to have been some unhappy event."

Here was a physician after my own heart. He was seeking for causes! He was not like the general run of doctors who said, "Find your cancer early." Why have cancer at all?

Let's read on: "In suggesting that a happy man is captain of his cells and master of his fate, and that he is thereby immune from certain diseases, I am sending up a provocative balloon that any real scientist could shoot down. Further, the word 'happiness' does not adequately describe the mood that I am striving to express."

Sir Heneage here shows himself to be cagey. He knows how cruel his brother doctors can be with regard to new ideas. So he protects himself by saying in effect . . . "I am only thinking out loud," but I am sure that deep down in his heart he really believes that happy people rarely get cancer.

Definition of Happiness

Finally Dr. Ogilvie says: "Happiness is a poor term for the state of spiritual ebullience that ensures happy government of the republic of the body, that repels the stress diseases, that can keep even cancer in check. Happiness is a pallid emotion. The word suggests groups of worthy people, too meek to have any vices, sitting on clouds and twanging harps. The emotion I wish to describe has no name, but the Greek word 'euphoria' and the modern slang 'one-upmanship' come near to it. It implies complete and rumbustious confidence, a jingoistic joy that is prepared for any trouble, perhaps hoping for it in the secure confidence that the conflict, should it come, will end in victory. It is the spirit that sustained Winston Churchill through the darkest days of the war, and that communicated itself to millions of his countrymen.

"The young man in love feels it. The surgical registrar feels it the day he gets his fellowship."

From the writing it sounds as if Dr. Ogilvie is a happy man in the ebullient, euphoristic sense. His is not the pale magenta type of happiness.

But one swallow does not make a summer. I couldn't prove a case just on this one observation, or prognosticate an axiom based on it. So I relegated it to some dustbin in the interior regions of my subconscious. I did quote him in our PREVENTION magazine, but without causing any ripples of excitement. Nothing came of it.

The Lancet

This was in 1959, but a few weeks ago I found in my files under date of 1955, another happening in this happiness-cancer category, which made a matching pair, and which gave me a decided thrill. In fact it "decided" me to write this book.

It was a letter that a doctor had written to the editor of *The Lancet*, my favorite medical journal, issue of May 21, 1955, as follows:

"Sir, — The subtitle, The Psychosomatic Disease, to Mr. Donaldson's article reminded me of a patient in her middle seventies who died recently of multiple secondaries from a carcinoma of the colon. Her illness had been slowly progressive and she had had an operation to relieve the obstructive aspect of it nine months previously. On her death bed, although she was unaware of the diagnosis, she was quite certain that she knew when this trouble with which she was dying had originated. This she stated quite categorically, was seven years ago when the minister of the church, which she had reverently cared for for many years and which she had many times scrubbed on her hands and knees, told her very gruffly to leave and not to come back. Thought of this incident grew in her mind until it was all consuming, in much the same way and at much the same time as the cancer developed and consumed her body.

"We know that suggestion can remove at least certain innocent growth on the skin and can cause 'burns' without heat. Is it possible that it can also cause abnormal growth in the body?"

R.N.R. Grant
Workington, (England)

Now we had two of a kind which made me feel that if I searched I would find more. So search I did, and found another article in *The Lancet* (1963) which, while it does not deal with cancer, will not hurt the general theme of this book.

This article represented a 5-year study made by 3 physicians connected with various medical institutions, which showed that grief is a factor in causing an excessive death rate among elderly widows during the first 6 months of their bereavement.

A potent factor, the doctors concluded, is the "desolation effect" immediately after the bereavement.

"The grief precipitated by the death is almost certainly associated with changes in the function of the endocrine (gland system) and nervous system," they added.

"Slowed movements, tears, and constipation cannot be the only body effects, they could scarcely fail to have secondary consequences for resistance of various illnesses." One of these various illnesses could be cancer.

Cancer in Negroes

According to my notes, some time in 1964, I was thinking about Ogilvie and his happiness theory when the thought struck me, that if happy people don't get cancer, or get less cancer, then Negroes should get less cancer than whites, for the Negro race is a happy race. True, there is their problem of segregation, but the Negro nature being what it is, I think a Negro sings just the same, and is not going to let segregation dampen his spirits as much as a similar problem would do to a white person.

At any rate, we looked up the cancer statistics and found them to be as follows:

	WHITE		NEGRO	
	Male	Female	Male	Female
1957	164.0	141.2	128.7	109.3
1958	161.9	139.6	125.6	100.1
1959	163.7	138.8	130.7	106.6
Average	163.2	139.8	128.3	105.3

The male whites get about 27 per cent more cancer than the Negroes. The female whites about 22 per cent more. Of course, there may be other factors, such as that the Negro gets more physical exercise because in the main he has to do manual work. There may also be differences in the diet. But who knows, perhaps some of the lesser amount of cancer is due to the Negro's generally happy temperament.

On the other hand, today with the Negro's constant demonstrations, and the whole racial tumult in which he is involved, the statistics with regard to his cancer incidence may undergo a change.

CHAPTER 2

Gardeners and Cancer

THINKING ABOUT Ogilvie, the charwoman, widowers and Negroes, made me go back to PREVENTION, issue of September, 1955, which was about 4 years before Ogilvie. I recalled that we had published the idea of a certain doctor to the effect that gardeners suffered less cancer than nongardeners.

I found the item: It was a letter a doctor had sent to the editor of the *Medical Journal of Australia,* and which appeared in the January 22, 1955 issue of that publication. Here it is:

"Sir: It is my clinical impression that patients who are active gardeners have a much greater host resistance to internal carcinoma (cancer) than do non-gardeners. Their survival period appears to be far greater in my experience. Whether this assumption is coincidental and false could be ascertained by practitioners working in city, suburban and country districts. May I, with respect, suggest this observation be made, and if established, submitted to the biochemists."

Yours, etc.,
Eric Goulston, M.D.
Sydney, December 20, 1954

I was terrifically excited about the item, and immediately got a letter off to Dr. Goulston, as follows:

Dear Dr. Goulston:

"I read your letter in the January 22, 1955 issue of the *Medical Journal of Australia* and I am wondering if you could give me more information about cancer and gardeners. We publish the magazine *Organic Gardening and Farming*, which represents Sir Albert Howard's idea of farming or gardening with nonchemical fertilizers."

Sincerely yours,
J. I. Rodale, Editor

Under the date of April 4, 1955, I received the following reply from Dr. Goulston:

Dear Mr. Rodale:

"Thank you for your letter concerning cancer and gardeners. All I can say is that I have noticed over the years that there seems to be a greater host resistance against cancer in patients who are suffering from this disease and who delve in the garden, than is the case with complete non-gardeners. This may be due to some anti-carcinogenic agent ingested from soils or from plants. We are trying to investigate this problem biochemically but haven't got very far, so that at present, it is only a clinical impression.

"I would be very interested to learn if any similar work is being done in the States. Your idea of not farming with chemical fertilizers, would make an interesting study for a surgeon in your district to investigate and compare the incidence of cancer there as with other centers.

"I would like to hear from you again. I hope to visit the States next year, and if in Pennsylvania, I should like to make your acquaintance."

Electricity and Magnetism

Dr. Goulston never visited me, nor did I know of any similar work done in this country. But I did have some gardening experience, and would like to express an opinion.

If you don't already know, I am the person who introduced the organic method of farming and gardening into the United States, publishing the monthly *Organic Gardening and Farming* which has about 350,000 subscribers. PREVENTION has over 400,000. I am the editor of both these publications.

I would think that gardeners get more exercise in the open air, thus oxygenating the body and causing it to function in a more efficient manner than that of a lethargic, nonactive person.

I have seen some cancer figures which showed that

rural folk get less cancer than city people, which could be because they garden more.

It is a known fact that the earth contains electricity and magnetism. In fact it has been said that the world is one big magnet. We know also that the body is an electrical power station, every cell being charged with electricity. Could it not be possible, therefore that in placing the hands in the soil, an electric circuit between the body and earth is completed, and that some of the ground electricity gently begins to course through the body, invigorating the latter? In other words, if a person gardens every day, is he or she receiving a healthful daily electrical treatment?

But isn't it quite possible that the average gardener is a happier person than a non-gardener? I have known many gardeners in my time and my general impression is that they are more or less of a happy group.

The gardener has his little world, away from the world. While he gardens he forgets his troubles, which makes him happier while he is gardening than when he is not gardening.

The gardener sees the miracle of creation, the growth from the seed to the harvested plant. He sees flowers spring up as if by magic, and if he gardens a hundred years he will never cease to marvel, nor to enjoy his flowers, his vegetables or his fruit.

But your non-gardener will find a dozen reasons why not to garden. He will sit around brooding while his neighbor is reveling in his little plant world, weeds and all.

A survey should be made to check on cancer cases

and whether they were gardeners. If there is a connection, then the Cancer Society could start a national publicity campaign to encourage people to go in for gardening.

CHAPTER 3

The Happy Hunzas

THE HUNZAS are a hardy race of people who inhabit the northern tip of India, and who are called the healthy Hunzas. They may also be called the happy Hunzas. Sir Robert McCarrison, a great English research physician, spent over 10 years with them and in 1921 lectured about them in the U.S. He delivered the 6th Mellon Lecture at the University of Pittsburgh.

McCarrison was amazed at the health and immunity record of the Hunzas, who, though surrounded on all sides by peoples afflicted with all kinds of degenerative and pestilential diseases, still did not contract any of them. In his Mellon Lecture he said, "They (the Hunzas) are unusually fertile and long-lived, and endowed with nervous systems of notable stability. Their longevity and fertility were, in the case of one of them, matters of such concern to the ruling chief that he took me to task for what he considered to be my ridiculous eagerness to prolong the lives of the ancients of his people, among whom were many of my patients. The operation for senile cataract appeared to him a waste of my economic opportunities, and he tentatively suggested instead the introduction of some form of lethal chamber, designed to remove from his realms those who by reason of their age and infirmity were no longer of use to the community."

So vibrant was the health of those Hunzas with whom McCarrison came into contact that he reported never having seen a case of asthenic dyspepsia, or gastric or duodenal ulcer, of appendicitis, mucous colitis or cancer. Cases of oversensitivity of the abdomen to nerve impressions, fatigue, anxiety or cold were completely unknown. The prime physiological purpose of the abdomen, as related to the sensation of hunger, constituted their only consciousness of this part of their anatomy. McCarrison concluded this part of his lecture by stating, "Indeed, their buoyant abdominal health has, since my return to the West, provided a remarkable contrast with the dyspeptic and colonic lamentations of our highly civilized communities."

Disposition of the Hunzas

Travelers who have lived and worked with the Hunzas are unanimous in praising their general charm, intelligence, and physical stamina. The Royal Geographical Society in a report in June, 1928, *Journal of the Royal Geographical Society*, Vol. LXXI, No. 6, said: "The Hunza men were with us two months, continuously on the move, over what is probably some of the worst country in the world for laden men. Always ready to turn their hand to anything, they were the most cheerful and willing set of men with whom we have ever traveled."

General Bruce, who climbed Mount Everest, said, that as slab-climbers the Hunzas were incomparable, besides being "most charming and perfectly companionable." One writer, R. C. F. Schomberg, commented, "It is quite the usual thing for a Hunza man to walk sixty miles at one stretch, up and down the face of precipices to do his business and return direct." This author passed through the Hunza country many times. He describes how his Hunza servant went after a stolen horse "and kept up the pursuit in drenching rain over mountains for nearly two days with bare feet." Schomberg also tells of seeing a Hunza in mid-winter make two holes in an ice-pond, repeatedly dive into one and come out at the other, with as much unconcern as a polar bear.

Sir Aurel Stein records a trip of 200 miles made on foot by a Hunza messenger, a journey that imposed the obstacle of crossing a mountain as high as Mont Blanc. The trip was accomplished in seven days and the messenger returned fresh-looking and untired, as if it had been a common, everyday occurrence. The word "tired" does not seem to exist in their lexicon. In the *Journal of the Royal Society of Arts* for January 2, 1925, Sir Robert McCarrison wrote: "The powers of endurance of these people are extraordinary; to see a man of this race throw off his scanty garments, revealing a figure which would delight the eye of a Rodin, and plunge into a glacier-fed river in the middle of the winter, as easily as most of us would take a tepid bath, is to realize that perfection of physique and great physical endurance are attainable on the simplest of foods, provided these be of the right kind."

All travelers who have been through Northern India are agreed that the Hunzukuts are uncommonly supple dancers and far superior mentally and physically to the neighboring peoples. They excel in grace, charm, intelligence, and in dancing. The tired American businessman has no counterpart in Hunza. In that country every man dances, from the prime minister down to the six-year-old boy. The Hunzas are overcharged with energy and dancing is a stabilizing influence.

It is not uncommon for Hunza coolies, after toiling heavily laden with packs up steep mountainsides all day, to indulge in wild dancing in the evening. In *Among the Karakoram Glaciers* Jenny Visser-Hooft (1926) vividly describes one such event:

"In the evening the jemindar came and asked whether the coolies might dance for us. We always found it a good sign that they had enough surplus energy to expend on such a strenuous form of amusement after a long and tiring march, and on this occasion it showed that their happy mood had not yet vanished. There were several enthusiastic performers, and the lack of an orchestra was made up by the audience, all joining in the chorus, repeating the refrain with tireless energy, clapping their hands to mark the rhythm, and instigating the dancers to fresh efforts. Akbar, one of the younger coolies, a slender lad of great strength and endurance, did a very fine sword dance, using two sticks, which he twirled about his head with amazing rapidity. He was the *Jeune premier* of the ballet.

"Then two men executed a dance together, moving round the circle behind each other, the last man imitating the leader's gestures with automatic precision, all the while chanting a monotonous refrain which the chorus of spectators repeated with gusto. One of the men presented a comical sight, stepping along coquettishly in a manner that would have befitted a dainty damsel but seemed quite inappropriate to a sturdy ruffian enveloped in a voluminous dirty choga, with his legs incased in clumsy, ragged Russian boots. Some of the dancers sprang high in the air, like leaping fauns, which must have been a tiring performance. There were different variations of dances, as each village has its own particular style. It was amusing to watch for a while, and even more so to note the men's pleasure in this simple merry-making. They all thoroughly enjoyed it."

As you can see, the Hunzas are a happy people and do not get cancer.

Nutrition

McCarrison attributes the fabulous health of the Hunzas mainly to their diet and to the way they raise their food. In his book *Nutrition and National Health* he says:

"I know of nothing so potent in maintaining good health in laboratory animals as perfectly constituted food: I know of nothing so potent in producing ill health as improperly constituted food. This too, is the experience of stockbreeders. Is man an exception to a rule so universally applicable to the higher animals?" To develop this point he embarked on an ingenious series of experiments with albino rats at Coonoor in 1927. At this time he was director of Nutrition Research for the entire country of India, an assignment which gave him worldwide recognition as an authority on nutrition.

He decided to find out if rats could be endowed with health equal to that enjoyed by the Hunzas through feeding the rodents on a similar diet. One group was, consequently, fed the diet upon which the Hunzukuts and other healthy people of Northern India, such as the Sikhs, Pathans and Mahrattas, subsist. On the other hand, another group of rats were fed the poor diet of the Southern India rice-eaters, the Bengali and Madrassi. In his aforementioned book, McCarrison referred to a nutritional authority, McCay, who twenty-five years before had written "As we pass from the Northwest region of the Punjab down the Gangetic Plain to the coast of Bengal, there is a gradual fall in the stature, body weight, stamina and efficiency of the people. In accordance with this decline in manly characteristics it is of the utmost significance that there is an accompanying gradual fall in the nutritive value of the dietaries." And so McCarrison found it.

A third group of rats was subjected to the diet of the lower classes of England, containing white bread, margarine, sweetened tea, a little boiled milk, cabbage and potatoes, tinned meats and jam. The results were startling. McCarrison described the first group as being *hunzarized.* "During the past two and a quarter years," he stated, "there has been no case of illness in this 'universe' of albino rats, no death from natural causes in the adult stock, and but for a few accidental deaths, no infantile mortality. Both clinically and at post-mortem examination this stock has been shown to be remarkably free from disease. The Bengali group of rats suffered from a wide variety of diseases which involved every organ of the body such as the nose, eyes, ears, heart, stomach, lungs, bladder, kidneys, intestines, the blood, glands, nerves and reproductive organs. In addition, they suffered from loss of hair, malformed and crooked spines, poor teeth, ulcers, boils and became vicious and irritable."

The "English" rats also developed most of these troubles. They were nervous and apt to bite their attendants; they lived unhappily together and by the sixtieth day of the experiment they began to kill and eat the weaker ones amongst them.

Please note the statement that with a poor diet the rats became vicious and irritable. They were not happy rats.

Victor Heiser, who wrote *You're the Doctor,* visited McCarrison when he was conducting his epoch-making feeding experiments with rats. He was astounded at what had become of this "English" group of ill-fed rats. "I approached the cage of one of the rats," he wrote, "expecting to find the usual peaceful laboratory animal. What I found was a pinch of fury and hate. As I came near, the rat lunged at me. He was spoiling for a fight. His whiskers bristled and his rough hair stood on end. He was the typical belligerent, touchy, pugnacious, malnourished lower-class Briton. I've met a number of them in London." Is malnutrition a factor in producing wars?

It is my contention that the deficient, fragmentized, refined modern diet is at the bottom of much crime today. The brain is not nourished properly. Thus there is confused thinking, and vicious behavior. Many of our juvenile delinquents will undoubtedly grow up to become cancer cases, and it won't be their fault. It will be the fault of those whose responsibility it is to teach them good nutrition but who are not doing so.

Going back to McCarrison's work, note his statement to the effect that in his decade of residence among the Hunzas he did not see a single case of cancer; that he found a high degree of longevity in these people. Note also the mention by visitors of the charm of the Hunzas.

CHAPTER 4

The Nagyri

COL. R. C. F. SCHOMBERG has employed significant words in his comparison of the Hunzukuts with the Nagyri. He said, "It is certainly difficult to understand how anyone, after having dealings with the Hunza people, could imagine that they had anything in common with their neighbors of Nagyr."

The Nagyri are darker than the Hunzukuts and outnumber them by a few thousands. They have vastly inferior physiques and are subject to many diseases, the most common of which is that of goitre and its companion evil, cretinism. Ella K. Maillart, in *Forbidden Journey*, describes even the Nagyr Mir's wife as suffering from goitre, and says, "So many of the inhabitants of those mountains were disfigured by goitre." Lorimer describes a jolly, cheerful Hunza crowd, "not a moron or a cretin among them: in a marked contrast to Nagyr, where both abound." The Hunza coolies employed by travelers and explorers have always been found to be superior to their Nagyri brethren.

Conway called the Nagyri "a low lot." Jenny Visser-Hooft said, "We were prepared for the cold, but we did not much like the look of our coolies (Nagyri). It seemed that they were the best the Wazir had been able to find for us, but they did not look very promising. They were of small stature and of much less favorable appearance than our Hunza coolies."

Mrs. Lorimer describes a visit to Nagyr and refers to the ungraciousness of the Mir's underlings, who "raised one difficulty after another about supplying our very modest needs." She makes allusion to the shrunkenness and frailness, to the rheumatism and heart condition of the Mir whose "people serve him ill," to the dirty and unswept resthouse in which they took up their quarters, and to "a general atmosphere of grudging incompetence." They passed "the miserable apology for a hospital, which contrasts ill with the well-built one at Aliabad, though the two Mirs got the same grant from the Government for the purpose of building them."

Schomberg adds another item to the list of evils that exist in Nagyr. He says, "My memories of Nagyr . . . have always been marred by the flies; there seem to be more there than elsewhere, and that is saying much! My Hunza man liked to see the flies, as they regarded them as a clear proof of the dirty habits of the Nagyri." Mrs. Lorimer corroborates this testimony.

Regarding the war with the British in 1891 Knight

emphasizes the apparent inferiority of the Nagyri. He says:

"The inhabitants of Passu (Hunza) discussed the recent war with us in a cheery way; they spoke of it as if it were some sort of *tamasha,* a merry little game that had been quite worth the playing. What tickled them immensely was the fact that by far the greater portion of the men who had been killed on their side had been Nagyri. 'The Nagyri did not want to fight,' said they, 'but our chiefs made them do so; and yet, lo! we Hunzas have escaped with very little loss, while hundreds of those other foolish fellows were shot.' "

Superiority of the Hunzas

The Nagyri, themselves, admit the superiority of the Hunzas, but attribute it to the fact that they live on the sunny side of the valley, which runs east and west. The Hunza mountainside looks to the south, and gets the maximum possible amount of sunshine, whereas the Nagyri live on the side of the river facing north. In the winter the sun penetrates little to their side, because of the extreme height of the mountains which screen them from the sunshine. For this reason Hunza is much warmer than Nagyr, where there is sometimes less than an hour's sunshine a day. It is generally held that because the Hunza land lies on the sunny side of the valley the people are more cheerful and healthy.

There can be no question that this is a prominent factor, but near them is another section where the Ishkomanis live and where they have maximum sunshine. Yet they, said McCarrison, "though living under apparently like conditions to their neighbors, were poor, undersized, undernourished creatures. There was plenty of land and water, but the Ishkomanis were too indolent to cultivate it with thoroughness, and the possibility of bad harvests was not enough to overcome their sloth. . . . They had no masons or carpenters or craftsmen in their country. Many of them showed signs of disease." The sun must be only one of the contributing factors that conspire to make of the Hunzas such a remarkable example of health and personality, but it is only a part of the story. Schomberg admits that the sun shines much less in Nagyr, even in the summertime, and for that reason their produce is inferior. He says further, "The people of Nagyr are poor husbandmen, believing rather in the kindness of Providence than in hard work, and their lovely fertile country owes but little to its owners."

The Hunza is a charming person, ever ready to greet you with a smile. The Nagyri will rarely accost you as you pass or give you a smile. Mrs. Lorimer brings this out graphically when she says:

"As we rode through Nagir and noted the dour looks of the Nagirkuts, the crouching, face-averted women, the absence of spontaneous 'good days' which brighten every Hunza chance encounter, the fact that when a Nagir prince was riding with us his passage was unmarked by any welcome or salute, our Hunza men would murmur with a grim satisfaction: 'Their caps are black, and their cloaks are black, and their mosques are black, and by Allah their hearts are black!' All travellers who have passed through the two adjacent states have noted the relative gloom of Nagir."

The cheeriness and geniality of the average Hunzukut is proverbial. Mrs. Lorimer says that there never was a people anywhere with such a gift for looking happy as the Hunzukuts. Their graciousness, good manners, contentedness, hospitality, lack of servility, aptitude for laughing and joking, and the pleasant relations which exist in the average Hunza household can be due to only one thing—health!

In 1927 Captain C. J. Morris explored the Hunza country and its glaciers, and in the following year made a report to the *Royal Geographical Society* in which he said, "These men were with us for just two months. During this time they were continuously on the move and over what is probably some of the worst country in the world for laden men. Always ready to turn their hand to anything, they were, I think, the most cheerful and willing set of men with whom I have ever travelled. . . . At the worst part of all we halted in order to help the porters across. They disdained our proffered assistance, however, and came over, climbing like cats, and with never a murmur at the hardships of this day's work."

Knight referred to them as "strongly-built men, with bold eyes and rather jovial expressions." General Bruce in 1928 in the *Proceedings of the Royal Geographical Society* said, "I found the Hunza people most charming and perfectly companionable." Buckle, in his *History of Civilization,* says, "It is proved by history, and especially by statistics, that human actions are governed by laws as fixed and regular as those which rule in the physical world. . . . Climate, soil, food, and the aspects of Nature are the principal causes of intellectual progress." The health, the spirit, the joviality, the intelligence of a people are what Buckle intimates in his term "human actions," and these actions are as closely linked up with soil, food, and climate as any two things could possibly be. But they all trace back to the soil and its maintenance. The Hunzukut is a more expert husbandman than the Nagyri.

Though the Nagyri have more land and much more water, they are less thorough in their methods of cultivation. The Nagyri side of the valley is more green and has more tree and shrub growth because the soil there is not made arid by the rays of the sun as it is on the Hunza mountainside. The Nagyr side compares favorably with the appearance of a Pennsylvania mountain. The Hunza looks like the Arizona desert hills. The Nagyri have a profusion of beautiful well-developed trees, but trees are scarce in Hunza. The crops and orchards of the Hunza seem less luxuriant than those of Nagyr.

But the Hunzukut is an adroit agriculturist as Lorimer shows:

"The fields were being reaped, and I marvelled at the neat, tidy rows in which the cut barley was laid out. Everything the Hunzukuts do is beautifully done, and their methods are in the greatest contrast to the slovenliness of Nagir; you notice this everywhere, down to the tiniest detail; it may be merely because water is scarcer and life harder that their fields are more scrupulously level, their walls more ingeniously perfect, their cut swathes more exactly aligned, but I incline to think that the cause lies deeper; in the difference of race and temperament already suggested."

We can adduce still another example: The Nagyri value highly the wool of the Hunza sheep which is far superior in quality to theirs, and yet they, themselves, have much more pasture land available for their sheep, which nevertheless yield an inferior wool. It is a mystery which can be solved only by disinterested scientific investigators who must examine the Hunza and Nagyr soils and all other factors and determine exactly what causes this difference. I say "disinterested," because there are some agronomists in this country who in their writings have expressed an open hostility to all organic composters. If left to them, they might want to introduce chemical fertilizers into the Hunza valley.

The Nagyri women are not allowed to be seen by a man. They will crouch down, turn their backs and cover their faces. Mrs. Lorimer while visiting their side of the river never saw a woman's face. When approached they will run for dear life. They wear unsightly dark bonnets which entirely cover their hair. Contrast this with the Hunzas, whose womenfolk are cheerful and go about without restrictions. They are as happy in their manner as the menfolk. They are rosy-cheeked and good-looking. Knight describes them as "really very pretty, having rosy complexions, good features and lovely eyes."

Actually the difference between these two peoples is that the agricultural practices of the Hunzas yield up healthier food. The Nagyri will burn manure as a fuel to keep warm, the Hunza will never do this. Every bit of manure goes into his soil and thus the plants have a higher mineral and vitamin content.

The fact that a Hunza is a more happy person than a Nagyri, along with the other evidence on this point contained in this book, must convince even skeptics that there *is* a relation between health and happiness.

CHAPTER 5

Roseto, Pennsylvania

PERHAPS YOU HAVE BEEN READING about a small town in Eastern Pennsylvania called Roseto, which has a very low rate of heart disease deaths (about one-half the national average), and where the people are very happy. This information was revealed by Dr. Stewart Wolf, head of the University of Oklahoma's Department of Medicine, in 1962. When the news hit the newspapers, the theme seemed to be that these Rosetans were a very happy people, and therefore they lived long, and with less heart trouble.

Roseto is a community of 1,600 inhabitants, practically all Italians, who "know how to get fun out of life." There seems to be a happier atmosphere here, says Dr. Wolf. In Roseto people enjoy themselves. They are vigorous, comfortable and generally happier than anywhere else in the U.S. They really live!

In the usual American community, people engage in a kind of rat race, Dr. Wolf observes.

"They don't have much emotional support from each other. Living is highly competitive—a constant keeping-up with the Joneses.

"Contrastingly, Roseto is a highly democratic town. Everyone has his place and appears to be pretty happy with what he has to do.

"Jobs people have are not much different from those in other communities, but social life is more pleasant."

As far as jobs are concerned the people work in the textile industry, many of the women working in shirt and blouse factories. Some of the men work in slate quarries. Others commute to Easton and Bethlehem to work in steel and other industries. Years ago, however, almost all the men worked in the slate quarries.

Here are the death statistics for Roseto and a few neighboring towns for 1961:

	Population 1960	*Number of Deaths*	*Rate per/1000*
Roseto	1,630	11	6.7
Nazareth	6,209	71	11.5
Stroudsburg	6,070	97	16
Bangor	5,766	64	11.1
Pen Argyl	3,693	63	17.1
Wind Gap	1,930	27	13.9

(The rate for the entire U.S. is 9.5)

The medical investigators are baffled since the Rosetans have more animal fat in their diets than most

Americans, which would discredit the theory that saturated fat intake and heart disease are connected. The Philadelphia *Sunday Bulletin* (January 27, 1963) referred to the borough of Roseto as probably the most overweight community in the nation (a fact that Rosetans considered exaggerated).

The *Bulletin* went on to trace the town's history. Founded about 73 years ago by immigrants from Roseto, Italy, it quickly became close-knit, because the newcomers were rejected by the older settlers of the area. Many of the newcomers were related. Forced together, they wove a web of mutual concern and friendship. Dr. Wolf said, "We found a happier atmosphere in Roseto than in most communities because people here like each other."

For several years, on and off, Dr. Wolf and his staff examined most of the adult population of the town, and their report of it appears in the June 8, 1964, issue of the *Journal of the A.M.A.*

The article speaks of the way the Rosetans seem to enjoy life, being gay, and boisterous, but unpretentious. They are simple, warm and very hospitable people. They were found to be mutually trusting, and without any criminal tendencies, there being very little crime in Roseto.

The article states that obesity and a generous consumption of calories, fat and wine were actually associated with a strikingly low death rate fom myocardial infarction, a form of heart attack.

To give an example of the comparison of this form of heart attack in Roseto with 4 other nearby towns, a table is given of the death rate from this condition per 100,000 of population, averaging the 7 years from 1955-1961, as follows:

Roseto	*157*
Nazareth	*603*
Bangor	*613*
Stroudsburg	*671*
East Stroudsburg	*405*

According to the article, the cholesterol in the Rosetans is about the same as in other Americans. The doctors state, therefore, that this is not a factor in producing the low Rosetan death rate.

As far as dietary habits are concerned, "a favorite dish, *prosciuto*, a pressed ham delicacy, has a rim of fat more than an inch thick and the Rosetans eat it whole without discarding the fat . . . cooking is done by most families with lard rather than olive oil . . . and most dipped their bread in the gravy to consume the whole dish."

The article winds up by saying that the reason for the low death rate from myocardial infarction in Roseto is not very clear, and is still to be determined.

Hill Walking

When the first account of the situation in Roseto appeared in the newspapers I read about it with avid interest, but I questioned the idea that they are living long because they are a very happy people. I recalled the case of the Hunzas of Northern India. They too are a very happy people, with practically no crime. But it has been shown that they are happy because they are healthy, and not healthy because they are happy. I decided it would be necessary for me to go to Roseto and see what I could observe.

It being only about 40 miles from Allentown, my wife and I went there in the summer of 1963, and we have been there several times since. The first thing that hit me was the fact that there are so many steep, hilly streets in this town. This has not been mentioned anywhere in the dozens of news items I have seen about Roseto, or in the *JAMA* article mentioned. But walking up and down hills from childhood can be a terrific factor in the health picture. And these older Italians brought the habit of walking from the old country.

Walking uphill increases the specific gravity of the tissues of the body, which enables the whole body, including the heart, to operate more efficiently. A high specific gravity means that the tissues are more compact. There is more weight to each cubic inch of body tissue.

Walking and exercising generally reduces the blood pressure and the pulse. I would suggest that in their continuing work, Dr. Wolf and his staff take specific gravity and blood pressure readings in the five towns. It may show a decided difference between Roseto and the other towns. I would suggest also a comparison of pulse readings in the five towns. Dr. Raymond Pearl of Johns Hopkins proved that on the average, the higher the pulse the shorter the life.

Talking about hill walking, there is a sanatorium in

Bad Nauheim, Germany, which specializes in heart cases. It makes use of three long hills, one with a 5 per cent grade, the second with a 10 per cent grade, and the third with a grade of 15 per cent. The patient is gradually conditioned until he can walk the 15 per cent grade with ease, and it has been found to strengthen the heart.

If these Rosetans did not walk these hills, they would be even more obese, their blood pressure and pulse would be higher, specific gravity lower, and their cholesterol still higher, for it is known that cholesterol is lowered by exercise. A high degree of obesity, on their high fat diet, with no exercise, would reduce their lifespan.

In one of the newspaper accounts about Roseto (Allentown, Pa. *Call*, October 6, 1963), is shown a picture of the contented face of Joseph Trilli, aged 94. The caption reads, "Enjoying good health, the nonagenarian can be seen taking his daily walk." The older Rosetans like to walk. I was talking to a grocer whose place is on top of a hill. He said that most of his customers walked up the hill two or three times a day to get their groceries. He said, "The older people walk, but the younger people, if they have to go five blocks, ride." The older citizens worked harder. Roseto was dug out of a chestnut forest by hand. They had no bulldozers.

Organic Method of Gardening

Point number two is something that I had a hunch about, as soon as I heard about these healthy Italians.

Most of them raised their own vegetables, and many of them kept chickens so they not only consumed fresh food, but most important of all, I found that very few people in Roseto used chemical fertilizers or poisonous insecticides. They were following the organic method of gardening without knowing it by name. It was a tradition with their people in the old country which they brought with them. This is a tradition-loving people as I could see from the names of the streets in the town—Garibaldi, Columbus, Dante, etc. In the old country, anyone who had even a pocket handkerchief-sized piece of land who didn't grow vegetables was akin to a renegade, and it is the same in the American Roseto. But neither place depended on chemicals.

I needn't go into the subject too deeply, but food raised organically has more vitamins and minerals than food grown with chemical fertilizers, although the *Journal of the A.M.A.* has violently attacked this idea. Then their writer has written articles so riddled with inaccuracies and omissions that it isn't even funny. We have published a booklet giving evidence only by physicians that organically raised food is more healthful than that raised by the usual chemical method.

My wife and I went from garden to garden—every house had one, and we saw only one that used a mild form of chemicals, but a neighbor told us that it was the case of an Italian woman married to an outsider. These people use manure as their fertilizer medium. Today the number of gardens has been reduced, unfortunately for Rosetans.

Nutrition of the Rosetans

So, we have here a people who move about in hilly streets, and who raise a good part of their food in their own backyards in a wholesome manner. Now, how about their diet generally?

I can refer to the tradition of breast-nursing which was brought from the old country. The medical statistics prove that people who have been breast-nursed for a considerable period are the healthier for it. The doctors should check the trend today among the young folks in Roseto. Are they keeping up this tradition? What is the incidence of breast-nursing in Roseto as compared to the four towns?

While on the subject of breast-nursing let's consider milk, and the part it plays in the Rosetan diet. It will be found that they drink far less milk than the people in the other four towns. The Italians drink wine and there is practically a complete absence of milk drinking, in the older people. On a trip to Rome and Palermo recently, I noted that milk is used so little compared to the U.S., that it is sold in tobacco shops.

I spoke to older people in Roseto. Several of them told me they never drank milk at all. The old generation even dipped bread in wine and fed it to babies. Today, I am told, this is no longer done. Babies get more store milk and eat boxed cereals.

The older people were more frugal. They wouldn't eat ice cream except on rare occasions. In other words their total consumption of dairy products is far less than that of the neighboring towns. Now if I had the space

I could give you 30 or 40 medical references to show that milk is *not* a healthful food for adults. It not only produces allergies in an enormous number of people, but recently it was found that children get nutritional anemia by the overconsumption of milk, and an article in *Nutrition Reviews* (April, 1963) stated that some athletic coaches found that milk-drinking impairs prolonged athletic performance. I can give you dozens of references indicting milk-drinking as the cause of various disease conditions.

But the most amazing thing of all is that excessive milk-drinking in children increases their stature. That is why our youth today are growing into giants, a condition which is not desirable. Very tall people do not live as long as shorter-statured ones.

In Dr. Wolf's article in the *JAMA* charts are given showing that the Rosetans are shorter in height. The Italians generally are very short people. So are the French. This is due to the fact that they drink very little milk, preferring wine. On my visits to Roseto I noticed how short the people were—much shorter than the people in the other four towns. But I did notice some very tall young Rosetan adults, who no doubt had been reading or were told that milk is a healthful food. They no doubt are also eating a lot of ice cream.

I recommend to Dr. Wolf that he study this milk factor, and that his staff make a thorough study of the medical literature on the subject to get at the truth about milk.

The Rosetans, old and young, do eat cheese, but as most Italians do, prefer the low-fat cheeses.

The bread favored by the Rosetans is the typical Italian white bread made locally with far fewer chemical additives in it. For example, it does not contain any anti-staling chemicals, will stay soft much longer. The fact of the matter is that in the diet of the average Rosetan there is much less of chemical additives. They don't patronize the T.V. dinner, consume very little of canned foods, and won't go for frozen beef. They want local butchers to dress it. Boloney is made in Roseto without using any sodium nitrate as a preservative. They consume more raw foods and fresh fruit. It is a custom from the old country. The medical people should attempt to compare the amount of chemical additives consumed in an average daily diet in the five towns.

Another aspect about their diet is covered in a letter to me from C. B. Axford of New York City. He says: "Can it be possible that the researcher—Dr. Stewart Wolf of the University of Oklahoma—missed the obvious reason? Out of my acquaintance with some Roseto folk, and their fare, I suggest you look into the relatively large amount of garlic which Rosetans consume. This is one great dietetic difference between Roseto and the neighboring towns with which Dr. Wolf attempted to compare it.

"How's about your making a little supplementary study and giving the facts to Dr. Wolf? Garlic's medicinal values are well known folk medicine among the Roseto oldsters."

American doctors don't think much of garlic but European researchers show that it can reduce high blood pressure, and is a natural antibiotic. Many opera stars eat garlic, claiming it prevents them from getting sore throats.

Then the wine of the Rosetans! The grapes for it are home grown. I saw garden after garden with their rows of grapevines, growing organically, without chemical fertilizers or poison sprays. The Rosetans make the wine themselves, using no chemical additives. The wine you buy has been treated with various chemical compounds for various purposes.

Again I say, the big thing with these Rosetans is that they get very little of the chemical additives which the average American has to ingest in his food every day.

Now, since they depend mainly on wine, the oldsters rarely drink soda pop or colas which have such a high sugar content. In the surrounding areas, however, large amounts of sugarized soda pop are consumed, and this is a point worth studying in connection with the Rosetan longevity and immunity to heart attacks, for the latest medical researches coming from England implicate sugar consumption rather than fats as a cause of heart attacks.

Sugar and Heart Attacks

Dr. John Yudkin, who is professor of nutrition and dietetics at the University of London, reported in *The Lancet* (July 4, 1964) on a study he had made in London hospitals, comparing patients with heart attacks or atherosclerotic conditions with a normal control group. He found that in every single case, the heart patients consumed at least twice as much sugar as those who had normal hearts and arteries.

In reporting this, he pointed out that in many years of intensive study, it has never been possible to prove there is any relationship between the fat that is eaten by an individual and cholesterol deposits in the arteries. Statistically, it can be shown that as a population becomes wealthier, heart disease increases, and many have believed this was because richer people eat more fat. But Dr. Yudkin has demonstrated that their consumption of sugar increases even more, and sugar is more likely responsible for heart trouble.

The average American consumes over 100 pounds of sugar a year. Can the University of Oklahoma doctors check and find out what is the annual sugar consumption in Roseto as between the oldsters and the new generation coming up?

I would like to say a few words about these youngsters in Roseto. They are not following the Italian ways with the intensity of their parents. They are eating more sweets, candies and refined foods. They don't go in as much for breast-nursing in their children. They drink milk and eat ice cream. Many of these young people own cars and get less exercise. They are taller and not as healthy as the older people. I was told they catch colds easily. I wonder if the average newly married youngsters arrange to do their own vegetable gardening.

Therefore, when the day of reckoning comes 30 or 40 years from now, will they live as long as the oldsters? Will Roseto be a medical experiment to show the effect on human health of the old and the new ways?

The Philadelphia *Sunday Bulletin*, January 27, 1963, had an article on Roseto with a big headline above it: "The Secret of Long Life in Roseto: Take it Easy, Eat, Get Fat, Be Happy." After having read my article you can see how wrong this advice is. If you want to live long, don't rush to Roseto. You can have a Roseto in your own backyard, where you can have an organic garden. And if you have a choice, pick a hilly area in which to live. Walk an hour a day and do calisthenics. Don't live in a ranch-type one-story house. Don't drink milk or eat dairy foods, cut out sugared soft drinks and refined foods, candies, pies, cakes, etc., and everything packaged or canned that contains chemical additives. Then you can look forward to living as long as do the Rosetans.

CHAPTER 6

Emotions May Have Cancer Link

IN *The Sunday Observer* of England, January 22, 1967, there is a short article with the above title, and I am reproducing it herewith:

"In the past 10 years research workers have been considering the possibility that the mind, and especially the individual's emotional life may play a part in causing cancer, a disease which in this country claims 72 victims a day.

"For example, Dr. David M. Kissen, director of the Psychosomatic Research Unit, Southern General Hospital, Glasgow, investigated 366 patients suffering from lung cancer. Though there was little difference in the number of cigarettes smoked by the cancer patients and the control group, there was a marked difference in the personalities of the individuals concerned.

"Dr. Kissen found that lung cancer patients tended to have poor emotional outlets. People who had adverse life situations and who repressed their feelings were more vulnerable to lung cancer than those who had good emotional outlets. Adverse life situations included disturbed marital relationships, poor relationships with parents and children, failure to gain promotion at work, and sexual difficulties.

"Strong supportive evidence for these findings was provided in a recent study undertaken by Drs. A. H. Schmale and H. P. Iker, of the Department of Psychiatry and Medicine at the University of Rochester Medical Centre, New York. Schmale and Iker selected 40 women who were known to have abnormal cells of the uterine cervix. They were interviewed the day after a definitive test for cancer had been made, but before the results of the test were known.

"The test took the form of an interview aimed at establishing the degree of hopelessness experienced by each patient. The interviewer then predicted on this basis whether or not cancer was likely to be present. This technique correctly identified eight out of 14 patients who had cancer, and 23 out of 26 who did not—an impressive result in statistical terms.

"Dr. Schmale says it is theoretically possible that the psychological reactions of these patients may be related to the preconscious or unconscious awareness of the presence of cancer in their own bodies. But it is equally possible that a life-history of endeavor coupled with a sense of hopelessness was a predisposing factor in the disease.

"None of these investigations implies that psychological factors alone are responsible for cancer, but they do suggest that there is some link between the disease and certain emotional states."

The above speaks for itself, and gives more evidence that cancer is less likely to strike happy people.

Dr. Denis Leigh

In the annual lecture of the Mental Health Research Fund, given in London, on November 1, 1966, Dr. Denis Leigh said the following, as reported in *The Lancet,* November 12, 1966:

"Epidemiological research had revealed illnesses in clusters related to life experience. Prisoners-of-war subjected to the harsh regimen of the Far East had more illness in later life than those who were in the European prison camps. Ex-prisoners of the Japanese six years later had twice the rates for cancer, heart disease, and suicide, and three times the rate for all forms of accident. These were not the diseases that would have been predicted. Inquiries in post-war Germany confirmed the pattern: Nazis dismissed from office had higher rates for all forms of illness than Nazis not dismissed."

Jack Ruby

The death of Jack Ruby, the slayer of Lee Harvey Oswald, fits into the pattern of this series. He died of cancer which induced a blood clot in his lungs. He had been a very unhappy man for a long time. Some people thought that his cancer was induced by feeding him cancer viruses, by mysterious interests that wanted him out of the way before another trial. But this is quite ridiculous.

Jack Ruby's death just adds another bit of evidence to our thesis that happy people rarely get cancer.

Ann Sheridan

Another case is that of the "Oomph Girl," red-haired Ann Sheridan who died of cancer in January, 1967, at the age of 52. She had always been a stormy petrel, was often suspended by the studios and would often go on strike for more money. Her life was a continuous struggle to go upward. She was married 3 times but never had a child. Ann Sheridan was too outgoing, too pushy.

There was a research at the Medical Research Council's Neuropsychiatric Research Unit, Carshalton, Surrey, England, which proved an earlier Swedish investigation that women who develop cancer are usually more extroverted, or outgoing in personality. In a study of 47 women, the results supported the idea that certain constitutional factors are associated with a predisposition of certain people to develop cancer. "Extraversion and other distinguishing factors may be related to physique and hormonal activity."

Our Experiment With Mice

In 1949, as president of the Soil and Health Foundation, I was associated with Dr. Ehrenfried Pfeiffer in an experiment in the feeding of mice at his laboratory at Threefold Farms, Spring Valley, N.Y., the results of which were reported in *Bulletin 2 of the Soil and Health Foundation,* dated November 1, 1949. The experiment was undertaken in order to find out whether the treatment of soil with organic materials or with commercial fertilizers would show a difference in the feeding and health values of products grown under such farming methods, and various groups of mice were fed by food raised by these different methods.

It was found that the death rate from fighting was distinctly higher in the chemical fertilizer group than in the organic one. There were more irritable and nervous mice in the chemical fertilizer group. I saw this for myself when I visited this experiment. The mice were kept six in a box and each box was divided into two rooms, because a mouse likes to sleep in one room and eat in another. In the partition between the two sections was a tiny door which was wide enough to permit one mouse at a time to walk through with comfort. When we opened up the chemically fertilized mouse box, that is, took off the top cover and let the light in, the mice became so frantic that they started to run. Two or three of them tried to go through the door at the same time, getting stuck and remaining there squealing and howling. But when we opened up the boxes in which the organically fed mice were kept, this did not happen. The mice continued nonchalantly about their business. It was interesting that the same thing happened time and again as we opened up the boxes. The chemically fed mice were invariably nervous while the organically fed ones were invariably relaxed.

Of the causes of death, stomach disorders were prevalent in the chemically fertilized group to an extent of about 16 per cent, but only about 3 per cent in the organic group. The results of this experiment showed that the survival rate of the organic group was markedly higher than that of the chemical fertilizer group: 32.63 per cent as against 21.38 per cent in the first generation. In another strain of mice the survival rate was 64.41 per cent in the organic group as against 35.39 per cent in the chemical group. Large litters were born to the organically fed mice.

Some time later an interesting experiment was performed. It is a known fact that certain chemicals when rubbed on the skin produce cancer. One of these chemicals was applied to the skin of all the mice. On that of the chemically fertilized fed group, cancer of the skin reached as high as 71 per cent, but in the organically fed group only 45 per cent contracted it.

The organically fed mice were a very happy group, but not so the chemically fed ones. This experiment shows that good nutrition is a significant factor in developing a happy spirit.

CHAPTER 7

Blood Sugar Affects Your Emotions

IN CONSIDERING what a person can do to prevent himself from falling into the type of chronic depression that has been characterized by various investigators as "hopelessness" or "despair," serious attention should be given to the question of whether it isn't possible to alter and improve the emotional state by simple means. As we will see in our study, large numbers of cancer patients before they were known to have contracted the disease had fallen into extremely depressed states, for very good reason connected with their own personalities and what life had done to them. Nevertheless, for every mother who devotes her life to her children and becomes utterly depressed when the children leave her, there are many other mothers in the same circumstance who survive the deprivation and manage to stay comparatively cheerful and very much alive.

In puzzling over what makes the difference in personalities, we have become convinced that the way a person eats has a great deal to do with it. And the most important element of all, it has come to seem, is the amount of sugar that is consumed in the daily diet.

There seems to be a direct connection between the excessive eating of sugar and many mental aberrations, prominent among which is severe recurring depression. The mechanism is a relatively simple one. Since an excess of sugar in the blood is a great danger, threatening areas of the brain with loss of consciousness and eventually loss of life, the metabolism reacts strenuously to an overdose of sugar. The pancreas secretes large quantities of insulin, which body chemical forces the sugar out of the bloodstream and into the tissues. One common result is overweight and another nearly or perhaps equally common, is mental fatigue and depression.

Low Blood Sugar

For an estimate of how common the condition of low blood sugar because of excessive sugar eating is, Dr. Sam Roberts in his book *Exhaustion* (Rodale Books, 1967) estimates that some 25,000,000 people in the United States suffer from hypoglycemia. Improper diet is not the only cause, but it is the cause in "approximately 70 per cent" of cases, according to the *Merck Manual of Diagnosis and Therapy*. Working out these figures, we can say that perhaps some 17,000,000 people in the United States are chronic depressives because they eat too much sugar.

In an article in *New Medical Materia* (August, 1962)

Cecelia Rosenfeld, M.D. dealt with the question of how hypoglycemia leads to emotional disturbances that can unnecessarily cause broken marriages. "One of the prime causes of marital discord—nutritional deficiency—is too often overlooked," she said.

"In my own practice, I have found that a surprising number of 'broken marriage' spouses suffered from a blood-sugar imbalance. Many of these husbands and wives showed symptoms of irritability, violent temper, abnormal sensitivity, and extreme fatigue. In most cases there was no evidence of organic disease."

One of the case histories cited by Dr. Rosenfeld was that of Mrs. R. L., a 34-year-old secretary, who "was referred to me by a psychoanalyst. Her symptoms included exhaustion, fatigue, exceedingly poor concentration, and chronic depression. As a result of these symptoms her home life had deteriorated and she was separated from her husband." From what we have already learned, we might well say that Mrs. R. L. showed the emotional pattern that might have been expected to lead to cancer. She was put on a nutritional regimen to regularize her blood sugar by Dr. Rosenfeld, and "four months later, improvement was so marked that Mrs. R. L. resumed post-graduate work which had been discontinued because of her condition. She is living with her husband again and both report that the marriage situation is harmonious."

Back in 1943 Joseph Wilder, M.D., of New York City reported in *The Nervous Child* (April, 1943) that a chronic state of low blood sugar produces mental symptoms in individuals which are not only characteristic of persons committing crimes but are also quite common among people we generally think of as "neurotic" or unbalanced or even just "difficult."

Here are some of the symptoms Dr. Wilder has found in patients suffering from low blood sugar: slowing of mental processes, dullness, difficulty in making even minor decisions, depression, anxiety, irritability, tendency to be negative, also physical symptoms like double vision, dizziness, changes in the voice texture, etc.

He reported that the qualities of mind most easily and earliest affected by low blood sugar are spontaneity and initiative. Mental and physical fatigue, apathy and indifference were mentioned by him as being common to this condition.

Quoting Dr. Wilder: "Apparently, too copious feeding of sugar may in the long run cause an overfunction of the islet cells of the pancreas and increase the tendency to hypoglycemia; on the other hand there are cases in which a diet extremely poor in carbohydrates and sugars may improve or even cure the condition."

In an address to the American Medical Association meeting in New York in 1957, Stephen P. Gyland, Sr., M.D., described hypoglycemia as the country's leading cause of suicides, schizophrenia, chronic fatigue and other effects of depressions.

Drs. Abram Hoffer and Humphry Osmond, who have developed a remarkably successful treatment for schizophrenia that depends largely on large doses of vitamin B_3, have recently come to recognize that hypoglycemia plays an important role in the mental disease. They have begun routinely treating their schizophrenic patients for hypoglycemia and Dr. Osmond reports that this is bringing him far better results than formerly. Allan A. Cott, M.D., a practicing psychiatrist, estimates that as many as 80 to 90 per cent of schizophrenic patients may suffer from relative hypoglycemia if not the chronic condition. Schizophrenia, of course, is a severe mental illness which is frequently characterized by periods of extreme depression.

Proper Diet

To overcome a condition of relative hypoglycemia (one caused by improper diet) soft drinks, ice cream, candy, sugar in any form and all foods containing sugar should be avoided like sin, which is precisely what they are. The only carbohydrates that should be eaten are whole, complex carbohydrates such as potatoes or corn, and very little of those. A high-protein diet is eaten with a normal amount of fat and plenty of green and leafy vegetables which are low in calories but high in vitamins and minerals. Dr. Roberts points out that supplements of the B complex vitamins and vitamin C are of extreme importance to help the patient regularize his blood sugar level. Brewer's yeast—the form of B complex recommended by Dr. Roberts—is also an especially high-grade source of specially nourished living protein. It is high-grade protein on which the body depends for an even flow of high energy that does not deplete the blood sugar and avoids the aftermath of exhaustion and depression that comes to sugar eaters. Brewer's yeast, therefore, is as perfect a supplement as one can find to aid in nullifying the effects of hypoglycemia and restoring one's energy and normal mentality. Dr. Roberts recommends that a teaspoon of it be taken between meals to help maintain the flow of energy throughout the day. He also recommends large amounts of vitamin C because this vitamin is directly concerned with the health of the adrenal gland. The derangement of the adrenal function is one of the common effects of hypoglycemia. To restore it to normal, Dr. Roberts considers vitamin C an absolute necessity.

Along with the vitamins recommended, Dr. Roberts states that his patients are forbidden to smoke or drink any alcoholic beverage. And he says it is most important to eat frequently in the course of the day and never allow yourself to get too hungry when fighting low blood sugar. Six times a day seems to be the number of eating periods that all agree will keep the blood glucose level just about where it should be without any perilous rises or falls, providing that every feeding is moderate and wise.

If you have ever had the experience of feeling tired, dragged out, unable to arouse interest in anything or energy enough to do very much, and then have taken a sweet and as if by magic have found yourself more cheerful, more alert and more energetic as well, then you understand the kind of transformation that can take place through a dietary change. The trouble with doing it through a sweet is that the effect quickly wears off and the eating of sweets only perpetuates the roller coaster ride your blood sugar takes. When you do it by eliminating all sugar from your diet, it takes a little longer—a few days or perhaps as long as a week. But you end up with your blood sugar at a proper level that encourages and permits you to be cheerful, alert and energetic all the time.

So eliminating sugar—every grain of sugar—from the diet is a very good rule for anybody who wants to stay happy and optimistic and avoid a pattern of despair and hopelessness.

Cancer and Blood Sugar

What has been presented here has been a physical way—dietary control—to improve the emotional state, deriving from the thesis that a very depressed emotional state leaves a person more prone to contract cancer. Remarkably, there has recently come to our attention a different kind of study that eliminates the middle step of emotional change but still draws a relationship between blood sugar abnormalities and the incidence of cancer. It was a study that came out of the Department of Oral Medicine at the University of Alabama Medical Center, Birmingham, Alabama, where Dr. E. Cheraskin has been doing some brilliant work in the study of early diagnostic signs through which later development of these diseases may be predicted. This particular study was reported to the A.M.A. Annual Convention in June, 1966.

The remarkable burden of his report was that a study of the carbohydrate metabolism—fundamentally of the way the system reacts to an overload of glucose—can give significant indications of whether or not the person being examined will develop cancer in the future.

What Professor Cheraskin and his associates did was to take advantage of the annual diabetes detection drive in Birmingham, as well as the availability of dental patients at the Department of Oral Medicine, to gather what most doctors would consider unrelated statistics and see if a correlation could be established between them. They studied two groups of dental patients, one comprising 120 and the other 170 persons, all of them well by normal medical criteria. 362 more people were examined in the course of the diabetes detection drive for 1964.

According to Dr. Cheraskin, "Several points warrant particular attention. Firstly, the higher the fasting blood glucose, the higher are the values for the rest of the tolerance pattern. Secondly, the higher the initial mean value, the less is the decline in blood glucose after 30 minutes. . . . Lastly, and most importantly, one can predict, within limits from *small* differences at the fasting level, the remainder of the glucose tolerance test patterns."

In other words, although a lengthy and cumbersome procedure, bothersome to the patient, is ordinarily used to determine the characteristics of the carbohydrate metabolism, it has been found that only the first step in this procedure is usually enough to give a clear indication of how the rest of the test is going to work out.

The figures for blood glucose were then compared to a different set of figures for the same groups, to check on the incidence of tumors. A correlation was found with age, as might have been expected, but also with the incidence of a high blood glucose level. In the oldest group, those above the age of 60, 22 per cent of those with the higher blood glucose levels had tumors as compared with only 6 per cent in the lower blood glucose group.

Checking back on the younger groups, the variation was not so sharp in the 30 to 59 year olds, but still existed in the ratio of 2 to 1. Below the age of 30 there were no tumors in either group.

Early Predictiveness

"The important point to be underscored is that small variations in blood glucose provide some measure of predictiveness," stated Dr. Cheraskin. What it comes down to is a strong indication that those whose metabolisms are unable to rapidly clear the blood of an excess of sugar are distinctly more likely to develop tumors in later age than those whose blood clearing mechanism is more efficient. Furthermore, a simple determination of the fasting blood sugar level may well be enough to unveil this entire pattern.

Dr. Cheraskin presented this report to the AMA, of course, in the hope that additional groups of doctors would be inspired to check it and either corroborate or refute it. It is, after all, a fantastically hopeful possibility to think that some day a doctor may be able to take a specimen of blood from a young man in perfect health and by determining the blood sugar level, know what probability there is that this healthy young man will develop cancer in 20 or 30 years. Given such a predictive tool, there is every possibility that the doctor could help his patient to avoid ever contracting cancer, or at the very least, would check him frequently enough to be able to make an early diagnosis.

It is the kind of tool many in the medical profession claim to have been searching and praying for. Has anyone followed up on the lead of Dr. Cheraskin and his associates?

We wonder.

A tendency to excessively high blood sugar is a problem that PREVENTION does not deal with as often as it is concerned with low blood sugar. That is because an excess of sugar in the blood is more a medical problem and is less amenable to correction by ordinary means such as dietary improvement. It should be pointed out here, however, that in its emotional effects, high blood sugar results in the same kind of derangements as does low. In fact, there is much evidence that most of the mental derangement occurs because of rapid changes in the blood sugar level, whether from high to low or from low to high; and the way to maintain a stable mentality is to maintain a stable level of blood sugar.

Another point to be considered is that people whose blood sugar level is unstable tend to be high at one time and low at another, making diabetes and hypoglycemia sometimes seem two different faces of the same coin. Elimination of sugar from the diet is fundamental to the treatment of both.

It all leads us to a still deeper question. Is it emotional depression caused by blood sugar abnormality that predisposes a person to contract cancer, or is it the abnormality of blood sugar regardless of the effect on the emotions? I do not think anyone can pretend to know the answer to that one. But either way, you can only benefit by deciding to give up sweets and all sugar-containing foods.

CHAPTER 8

Personality and the Thyroid

IN CONTINUING THIS STUDY of the relationship between cancer and the emotions, it is certainly appropriate to ask whether it is possible to influence the kind of patterns into which our personalities fall. The characteristics of the cancer-prone personality, such as alienation, hostility, hopelessness, and lack of focus or objective, are psychiatric classifications that a strictly medical man might well translate into the single word —depression. And considering the problem as simply one of depression might be a very helpful thing to do.

If you see that a person feels useless and unwanted, and want to change that feeling, you may think of elaborate and subtle arguments to prove that it isn't so. If you try using the arguments in a discussion, 999 times out of a thousand you will find that they make no effect. Suppose, on the other hand, that the doctor simply considers the attitude a depression and treats it with a euphoric drug like benzedrine. The drug alters the physical aspects of the depression—the hormone secretions, the heartbeat, the enzyme production. And with these alterations in the physical state, the patient actually thinks differently. He may, for instance, wonder why he felt so alone and isolated when there are so many nice, friendly people in the world. It is a fact that, by altering his physical state in very slight ways, you have not only altered his emotional responses but also what he thinks.

The trouble with using drugs for such a purpose, of course, is that the system quickly grows accustomed to them and requires stronger and stronger dosages; that the drugs themselves are toxic and damaging to the health in every case; and that such drugs are habit forming, in effect substituting the illness of addiction for another illness of depression. But the temporary success these drugs demonstrate in eliminating mental depression, simply by altering the physically depressed state, gives us an indication of what may well be the simplest, most direct and most successful way of avoiding falling into the habits of thought and personality that contribute or even lead to cancer. Keep the body healthy and the thought processes will be cheerful and healthy as well.

The influence of the blood sugar level in this respect has already been discussed. Low blood sugar—hypoglycemia—which is estimated authoritatively to afflict perhaps 25 million Americans, must certainly be the chief physical cause of depression and emotional despair. The avoidance of sugar in the diet and of all rich carbohydrate foods that overstimulate the pancreas into excessive production of insulin constitutes the basic answer to low blood sugar and the emotional difficulties it creates. But there are other measures as well that can benefit the health of the nervous system and therefore the health and clarity of the mentality, without posing any of the risks of the dangerous euphoric or tranquilizer drugs.

Mental Health and the Thyroid

One extremely important aspect of the fight against mental depression is the health of the thyroid gland. By controlling the rate at which the body oxidizes and produces energy, the thyroid has an enormous effect on the blood sugar level, and thus on the mentality. A healthy thyroid functioning at the proper level is just about indispensable for a healthy mind and personality.

At the Second International Congress for Psychiatry, Zurich, Switzerland (September 1-7, 1957) Nathan Masor, M.D. of New York City delivered a paper on the treatment of mental disease with the use of thyroid hormones, vitamins, and a diet specific to each patient's problem, usually of high protein content. These cases were selected from among hundreds in whom he had achieved favorable results.

Quoting from Dr. Masor's paper: "All patients treated . . . were acutely disturbed. They had been thoroughly processed in physical, x-ray, and laboratory examinations to insure that the conditions for which they were treated were (diagnosed as) solely psychiatric in nature. In every case there was a deterioration of personality, with element of affect (emotion) holding sway over the intellectual processes. . . ."

The medications used were a thyroid hormone, vitamin C, and vitamins of the B-complex—namely, thiamine chloride, riboflavin, and niacinamide, which are known as oxytropic elements (improving the transport of oxygen to the brain through complex enzyme reactions). Another compound consisting of *laevo thyroxin,* which is the natural hormone of the thyroid gland, and vitamin B_{12}, by injection, were the other medicaments used.

Here is one of Dr. Masor's case histories:

M. D., married, age 47, a woman whose tenseness is reflected in anxious fancies, rapid speech and tremulousness. Chief complaint over many years' standing was "nervous stomach." There was difficulty in concentration and she became very unsocial. Gastrointestinal x-ray series and other tests were negative. Multiplicity of other complaints, from chest pains to vertigo were present. She had previously been given a great deal of sedatives, different physicians, and a series of 14 shock treatments, with no lasting beneficial effects. She could not finish a day's work due to exhaustion. Insomnia was another prominent complaint. It took only five weekly injections of the thyroid hormone and B_{12} and the oral medication, starting in March, 1957, to effect a virtual reversal of the symptoms. There was a complete eradication of the stomach complaints, the state of exhaustion and the side complaints, and she states that she has never felt as emotionally secure as within the five weeks of treatment, with improvement starting after the third week.

All of Dr. Masor's cases followed the same pattern. Patients who had been subjected to a thorough differential diagnosis and whose problems were considered completely emotional and mental responded to increased thyroid hormone and vitamins that are necessary to the health of the nervous system.

A well-functioning thyroid is necessary because the secretions from this gland help the oxygen to be transported through the body. Drs. Danziger and Kindwall (*Diseases of the Nervous System*, August, 1948) stated that all mental disorders are symptoms of *anoxia* (oxygen deficiency), and in working with a series of 19 psychotic (insane) patients, they cured the deficiency by feeding them large doses of thyroid extract, and thus cleared up the psychosis.

They could have speeded up results if they had given their patients vitamins B and E, which are associated in maintaining the oxygenation of the body.

So, if you want to stay mentally healthy, look to the health of your thyroid. Of course, there are other causes of mental disease, but the under-active thyroid is a prominent one.

Now, how do we *maintain* a healthy thyroid? I think the first rule is to be generally healthy—a sound thyroid in a sound body! We must, therefore, be health conscious. Secondly, we must be sure of our iodine supply. All sea foods are rich in iodine. There are limited amounts in eggs, meats, vegetables, nuts, etc., but the best source is in kelp tablets. Two or three kelp tablets a day and you can forget about your iodine needs.

Aspirin has an immediate anti-thyroid action, says *The Journal of Endocrinology* (Nov., 1953), and low thyroid action is often the result of its use. In other words, the taking of aspirin by some people could cause mental symptoms. Avoid it.

In *The Journal of the A.M.A.* (Nov. 23, 1957), Dr. Arnold S. Jackson wrote that "the most important single factor responsible for symptoms of thyroid disturbance in 228 patients he observed was the over-indulgence in the use of stimulants—coffee, tea, and nicotine." Many of these patients smoked two or three packs of cigarettes a day, and drank from five to thirty cups of coffee each day!

There is a story about a girl called "Kathy" which is described in a book by that name, published in 1957 by E. P. Dutton Company. Kathy was a young girl who changed with alarming rapidity from a normal healthy child to a shadow. Her weight steadily dropped. Her good spirits and energy simply disappeared and she suffered from a frustrating inability to keep warm. One doctor after another was consulted, and each was forced to admit that he could find nothing wrong with Kathy. As a last resort, the child was taken to a psychiatrist who declared that she was suffering from psychosis and should be sent to a mental hospital.

Almost by accident, shortly thereafter, she happened to be in the office of an M.D. who decided to test the operation of her thyroid gland. He found it dangerously deficient, and gave her a thyroxin preparation to supplement the short supply in her body. In a matter of hours, her condition was noticeably improved. In a few weeks her terrible ordeal was over and she was back at school, a perfectly normal girl. Without the alertness of this M.D., Kathy might have been condemned to years of confinement in a mental institution, and eventually, to a premature death.

In *The Canadian Medical Association Journal* (Dec. 15, 1956), Drs. Ferguson and Rayport noted that the thyroid is known to have a direct connection with the central nervous system of the body. In a news release from the Lehigh County (Pa.) Medical Society, in the *Allentown Morning Call* (Jan. 2, 1958), it is stated that an emotionally distraught person may go to a psychiatrist, thinking he has mental trouble, when his real problem is an under-active thyroid gland. And, in the *New York Times* of Nov. 8, 1959 it was stated that at Cornell, based on researches extending over three years, it was reported that certain patients with serious mental illnesses are abnormal in the way their bodies use thyroid hormones. So, we are pretty sure of our ground when we say that, given a healthy thyroid, there is less chance of becoming mentally depressed than where there is a deranged thyroid metabolism.

This does not mean that a thyroid preparation should be used indiscriminately, or ever without medical supervision. What it does mean is that a basic step in trying to eradicate mental depression is a basal metabolism test to check on the level of thyroid function.

Thyroid hormone is about as natural as a drug can get. It is a hormone that is naturally produced in the human system. For medical use, it is obtained from the thyroid glands of animals, nor can it be synthesized in a chemical laboratory. It is a natural stimulant of the basal metabolism, the rate at which food is used up by the body.

Because it has this unique ability, and does not add anything unnatural to the system, thyroid extract and hormone have long been considered potentially valuable tools of medicine. Its use, however, definitely requires simultaneous vitamin administration to prevent side-effects.

Thyroid extract alone has been found to cause an accelerated, fluttering heartbeat. It has induced toxic reactions. It has been found so unpredictable in its effects, that most doctors will go to great lengths to avoid using it.

The way to use it is to add large quantities of vitamin C and vitamin B complex to the treatment. Almost like a miracle, these vitamins eliminate every undesirable effect of the thyroid hormone, returning to doctors what potentially should be one of their most useful tools.

One place where this comparatively natural drug is once again being used, with renewed enthusiasm, is the Vascular Research Foundation in New York. Its director, Murray Israel, M.D., reports successful control of high blood pressure and hardening of the arteries with this thyroid-vitamin combination. A generation ago thyroid hormone was condemned especially in cases of hardening of the arteries. B vitamins and vitamin C experimentally added to the thyroid extract by Dr. Israel had an almost miraculous effect. His results were reported to an A.M.A. meeting in Denver, Colorado, in November, 1963. They not only eliminated the alarming and dangerous side-effects but in high enough quantities they prevented the characteristic development of vitamin shortages which stem from the administration of the thyroid hormone.

"It is most essential that these protective vitamins be given in standard amounts along with the thyroid extract," Dr. Israel said. "To put it another way, thyroid extract cannot be successfully or safely administered continuously without them."

Others now using the same therapy with the same success include the famed Brusch Medical Center of Boston, and the noted Dr. Broda Barnes of the University of Colorado.

For a day to day health program, we believe the lesson to be drawn is the value of large amounts of natural vitamin C and B complex in the daily diet. Seeing how they work hand in hand with the thyroid, we would guess that large daily amounts of brewer's yeast, desiccated liver, wheat germ, rose hips and acerola might be just what is needed to keep the thyroid from ever developing a disorder in the first place.

CHAPTER 9

Pinning Down the Cancer Personality

SOMETIMES, WHEN DEALING WITH WRITINGS in the area of psychology, we have to stop and ask ourselves whether we really understand the terms describing personality that are used by psychologists. Their writings are not on the same level as medical literature. When a doctor refers to a tooth, a hangnail or a heart, we know exactly what he is talking about. Even if he uses an unfamiliar term such as, for example, *Escherichia coli*, all we have to do is to go to the dictionary to learn that it is a type of bacteria with a precise shape that can be seen under the microscope and identified. But it is a very different matter when a psychologist refers to an "inhibited" or a "repressed" personality.

Just what do these words mean?

Even if we think we understand them, it is worthwhile checking on our understanding because so many people have written so much nonsense in the newspapers and magazines, using such terms loosely and very often without understanding themselves just what their terms mean. A lot of vulgar misconceptions have grown up, consequently. When we talk of an "inhibited" person, the first idea that leaps to mind is someone who does not permit himself to enjoy sex relations. But to a professional, inhibition may deal much more commonly and much more significantly with a person's inability to get angry when he is provoked, and a man may have a great relationship with his wife and still be inhibited as a psychologist sees him.

Thus it is appropriate to try to clarify for ourselves precisely which kind of people we are talking about when we quote the findings of various studies to the effect that those who develop cancer are characterized by repression and denial. Does this mean that these are people who won't spend the price of a new dress or suit? Are they abstemious in their eating habits or finicky about body odors or just what are they really like?

Cancer-Prone Personality

A descriptive paragraph would not tell us very much, since it would raise the same problem of just how to understand the words that are used. But there is a much clearer method that was used by Claus Bahne Bahnson and Marjorie Brooks Bahnson of the Jefferson Medical College in Philadelphia in a study they made.

They conducted interviews with "24 patients, male and female, with different types and sites of cancer, from different walks of life, of different ages from 16 to 73, and living in different cities on the East Coast." Among other interview elements, these patients were asked long series of what are known as "forced-choice" interview questions. Such questions require that a statement be answered as either true or false, or in some cases that the one answering agrees or disagrees with the statement. Many such questions evoked such a random scattering of answers that they could be seen to have no particular significance. In some cases, however, there was a remarkable degree of uniformity in the way the cancer patients answered a particular question.

All such questions were listed by Bahnson and Bahnson, with the result that we are able to get a much clearer picture of the cancer-prone personality from the uniform attitudes of such personalities as reflected in their answers.

Here is one group of questions, and you will probably be as surprised as I was at how uniform the responses were and the specific type of personality they indicated.

	Answers	
	True	*False*
1. I was often sick to my stomach.	2	23
2. I could not keep my mind on any one thing.	3	22
3. I had periods of such great restlessness that I could not sit long in a chair.	4	21

4. My feelings were hurt easier than most people's.	3	22
5. A clear memory of my dreams often stayed with me for days.	4	21
6. My wife was not satisfied with my accomplishments in life.	4	21
7. At times I felt that I was going to crack up.	2	23
8. I can remember "playing sick" to get out of something.	1	24
9. I often had upsetting nightmares.	3	21
10. I felt hungry almost all the time.	2	23
11. When I went out, I usually preferred to go out by myself.	3	21
12. No one really understood me.	1	23
13. I often felt alone in the world.	3	22
14. Nothing turned out right for me.	3	22

Bahnson and Bahnson pointed out in reporting their study to the New York Academy of Sciences in 1965 that such uniform responses—far more uniform than were found in the responses of a control group of healthy people—could not be taken as representing the actual truth, but rather what these sick people wanted the truth to be. ". . . The cancer patients very definitely show a massive denial of all that can be embarrassing or is viewed as socially undesirable." In other words, these people were found to be socially conformist to such an exaggerated degree that even the mildest personality manifestation, such as having nightmares, that they thought other people might frown upon or consider queer, was immediately and unequivocally denied.

Not only were these cancer patients found to be unusually conformist, though, but it was also found that nearly uniformly their social attitudes depicted extreme conservatism and rectitude. These were the kind of people who would be pillars of whichever church they belonged to, dutiful hardworking employees, and more than a little stodgy—the kind of people who make others wonder what really goes on behind that mask of model behavior. Here are six typical questions which were answered with a startling uniformity.

	Answers	
	Agree	*Disagree*
1. Obedience and respect for authority are the most important virtues children should have.	22	2
2. Life is a serious business.	23	1
3. Honesty brings its own reward.	23	1
4. It is a wonderful feeling to sit surrounded by one's possessions.	18	6
5. Most people have a secret burden or cross to bear.	18	6
6. Most people are more nervous than appears on the surface.	21	3

Thus we began to get a picture of what it means in specific detail when earlier studies we have discussed have indicated that the cancer-prone temperment is repressed or inhibited or, what took us by surprise, extroverted. The repression is of behavior or even thoughts that it is felt would not be approved by one's parents in the first place or by society in general. The inhibition is no longer against sexual enjoyment which these days is hardly disapproved in the most conservative social circles, but rather against any type of behavior that might bring conflict with another person or people. And the extroversion is a technique of not feeling anti-social impulses by never examining oneself closely enough to be aware of them.

Another question used by Bahnson and Bahnson to define this special type of personality was: "When something makes you really angry which of the following are you likely to do?" The patient being questioned was presented with 15 different anger responses and asked whether he used each of these responses often, sometimes or never. The grouping of the answers was highly revealing.

Only four of the group replied that they would strike back when angered, while nine asserted that they never strike back and 10 more were in between. Only three admitted to such a violent response as swearing, kicking or throwing things. While 23 conceded that getting angry could make them shake or tremble with rage, all but four asserted that they tried to keep their anger to themselves as long as possible. Nineteen asserted that they respond to anger by trying to think about more pleasant things, and 21 granted that they had a tendency to apologize even though they felt they were right.

Thus, through these questions evoking specific situations, we get a very clear picture indeed of the kind of person who may be said to have a disposition toward contracting cancer. In a sense he might be said to have never grown up because, as an adult, he is still responding to the problems of his adult life in the same way he used to respond to the problems of family life as a child. When a father gets angry a child does not try to strike back and suppresses the anger with which he naturally reacts. And this type of response is necessary and wholesome for the child whose greatest need, after all, is for the authority of his parents to discipline him, to teach him how to behave, and to keep him out of trouble. Even though it evokes an instinctive resentment, authority to a child is the source of his security and happiness. But as he grows older his personality should also be maturing, relying only on itself for authority and security, and able to express its mature needs and desires.

The adult who has never outgrown his childhood ways of reacting to a challenge is least likely to be aware of unhappiness and yet is most likely to be intrinsically a person who feels unexpressed and unfulfilled—an unhappy person.

Bahnson and Bahnson stated it like this:

"A study of the unstructured interviews with our cancer patients reveals that they all had experienced very close attachments to a parent or parent substitute early in life. Apparently, they had not been able to transcend genuinely the early dependency of their childhood, although in some cases they had been able to function adequately on the basis of reaction formation and over-compensation. However, in those cases, this compensatory way of dealing with the unsolved dependency needs had collapsed from one to two years prior to clinical onset of the malignancy. For most of the other patients unsatisfactory resolutions of early developmental problems had resulted in relationships during adult life which repeated the dependent childhood patterns. This solution, in turn, gave rise to severe conflicts with which the patients tried to cope by denying and repressing them, sometimes with success over long periods of time. This strategy resulted in a continual constriction of their life pattern and led them into more and more narrow, rigid, and barren terms of existence, until they regressed to living only in terms of the most essential and narrow day-to-day routine. They then lived an emotionally frustrated, depleted, empty and barren life, with ever decreasing interpersonal stimulation and interaction, and with dwindling self-insight and self-communication. It was as if they lived two lives: one formal, realistic, and common sense oriented, filling a social and family role with near perfection, but with another wounded and despairing self, existing independently and unrelated to the conscious and social self, thirsting for affection, warmth and personal creativity. Strikingly, from a clinical viewpoint, no communication whatever seemed to exist between these two 'selves.' A split and a role reversal, so to say, had taken place between primary and secondary process functioning. The regenerative drive seemed to have taken off on its own, having deprived the secondary process activities from the fuel which otherwise might have fired and intensified every day interpersonal life. Now it was closed off and went its own way.

"The theoretical points which have emerged from the clinical studies of our cancer patients thus are: (1) that underlying dependency and affectual needs remain infantile, (2) that serious frustrations result in narcissistic regression and re-organization, and (3) that due to repression and denial, available energy potentials under the reign of this self-propagating narcissism are retained on the primary process level, uncommunicable through the social self which atrophies and follows a bleak, repetitive routine."

CHAPTER 10

Are Suicide and Cancer Related?

ONE OF THE LEADING FIGURES in the field of study of the relations between psychosomatic factors and cancer is Lawrence LeShan, Ph.D. The medical records are full of his work, much of which we will discuss in this book as we go along.

At this time we will look into an article by him, entitled "Cancer Mortality Rate," with the subheading, "Some Statistical Evidence of the Effect of Psychological Factors." (*Archives of General Psychiatry*, May, 1962.)

LeShan names many of the doctors who are working in their field (Kewal, Petscke, Greens, etc.) who have found a "certain life-history pattern in a statistically significant larger percentage of examined cancer patients than of equated controls."

He says, "One particular aspect of these life history

patterns has been the finding of an underlying emotional orientation which can be described as a bleak and hopeless despair about ever achieving any real satisfactions or meaning in life, apparently existing prior to the first noted signs of the neoplasm (cancer)."

This has been known for a long time, says LeShan, and is especially true of the cancer patient who does not respond to medical intervention. He has made the unconscious decision to die. This decision is made at deeply unconscious levels of personality, and death follows in a manner determined by the genetic, biochemical, psychological and environmental factors peculiar to the patient.

He mentions a Dr. Jores who "agrees with the other studies that specific objective *events* (such as permanent loss of an important relationship) whose statistical frequency is influenced by socio-economic changes, play a large part in the development of such an orientation."

LeShan got the idea that since suicides are based on a similar principle (social and socio-economic factors which affect the psychological status of individuals), "if a relationship could be found to exist between the yearly variations in the suicide mortality rate and the yearly variations in the cancer mortality rate" it would strengthen the case for the importance of psychological factors in cancer mortality.

Data were taken from the U.S. Census (Vital Statistics, Special Reports, of the Department of Health, Education and Welfare) and a study was made.

It was found that there did exist a definite relationship between the suicide mortality rate and the cancer mortality rate in the U.S. for the years 1914 to 1953.

The detailed figures are very complicated and will not be discussed here. LeShan summarizes: "It seems to indicate that factors which operate through psychological channels have a marked effect on the yearly variations in the cancer mortality rates."

Dr. J. Robert Oppenheimer

On February 18, 1967, Dr. J. Robert Oppenheimer died of cancer. As you know, Dr. Oppenheimer was the genius who pioneered the development of the atom bomb. He was 62 years old.

Since 1954 Oppenheimer was in "the doghouse," and was denied access to secret documents by the Atomic Energy Commission.

He was thrown out of the ranks of acceptable scientists because of alleged association with Communists in the 1930's and early 1940's while he was teaching at Berkeley.

Oppenheimer was a gentle person, and his public disgrace in 1954 no doubt began to eat into his inner consciousness, (his soul I was going to say).

President John F. Kennedy tried to restore Oppenheimer to public honor, and in 1963 President Johnson awarded him the $50,000 Enrico Fermi award, "for outstanding contributions to theoretical physics, and for his scientific and administrative leadership," but it was too late. This was merely a little salve to heal the surface. But underneath the cancer had already formed.

Dr. Hans-Joachim F. Baltrusch

In the *Journal for Psychosomatic Medicine* (Gotlinger) October-December, 1963, Dr. Baltrusch has published a comprehensive study of the field of psychosomatic research in cancer. I will quote a few excerpts:

"Modern technology has developed faster than the ability of humans to adapt themselves biologically and socially to altered living conditions. This leads to people suffering and dying more and more frequently from diseases which, in the last analysis, are due to a condition of tension between the single individual and his group, between his personal and social environment, or which are brought about by the activity of the person."

As he goes along Dr. Baltrusch gives names of doctors who have written on this subject. Later, Dr. Baltrusch says:

"Although there are an abundance of references, observations, and organized investigations from the earliest times to the present day which all point to the fact that there is a connection between psychosocial factors such as 'negative emotions,' anxiety, sorrow, depression and melancholia, personal catastrophes, and drastic situations in life—between all these and the occurrence of neoplasms (cancer), up to now this state of affairs has been almost completely neglected by medicine."

Again, "While children and young people are fulfilled with the task of finding themselves, the aging individual is exposed to the increasing danger of losses of objects, such as the death of the spouse, the children becoming independent, giving up the occupation, and the disappearance of sexuality. With the feeling of the evident reduction of his own physical and creative powers, rejected by his environment and society, this individual easily becomes the prey of geriatric diseases, cancer also being among them."

Near the end of his article, Dr. Baltrusch suggests that in the treatment of cancer, its psychosomatic aspects must be considered, that in many cases there is a failure in radium and chemical therapy because the disease was psychosomatically caused, and the cure should therefore be attempted along psychosomatic lines. He speaks of psychotherapeutic procedures—a strength of spirit must be induced which fortifies the resistance of the patient against cancer.

He says that "To my knowledge, with the exception of LeShan and Renneker, no serious attempts of psychotherapy in cancer patients have been undertaken up to now."

I have tried to figure out in my mind what would be the psychotherapy of cancer. I would imagine that a thorough case history of the patient be taken by a specialist who is expert in this field.

Fortified with this information the doctor can show the patient what has caused the disease, and urge him to change his frame of mind, so as to neutralize that cause.

Baltrusch says that there already have been successes resulting from psychotherapeutic measures.

I can see a new kind of cancer ward in a hospital with an effort made to make the patient happy. There would be live music, comedic pantomimes, the singing of comic songs, lectures on how to be happy, etc. The waves from live music will penetrate the patient's body and perhaps be one of the means of reversing the wild growth of the cells.

CHAPTER 11

Dr. Gotthard Booth's Writings

THERE IS A MAGAZINE called *Pastoral Psychology* which, as the name indicates, deals with psychological problems that fall upon ministers and priests. There is a particular article in the February, 1966 issue, entitled "The Cancer Patient and the Minister," by Gotthard Booth, M.D., which will be found very interesting to my readers. Dr. Booth is a member of the Committee on Medicine and Religion of the American Medical Association. I will quote the first paragraph in this article:

"In recent years the medical profession has become increasingly aware of the fact that the development of cancer is influenced, from the beginning to the end, by psychological factors. The minister, who is faced so often with cancer patients in need of pastoral help, can be most effective if he knows something about the nature of the personality problems which are specifically relevant in malignancies."

But for a long time, says Dr. Booth, there was strong resistance from medical men and from the lay public against psychosomatic research in cancer.

It took Dr. Booth 15 years to study the subject, to fight the resistance and finally to come out into the open with thoughts about his work. He says, "The mounting seriousness of the cancer problem has now begun to reduce the resistance against the psychological approach."

Cancer and Personal Relationships

I will give a few pertinent excerpts of Dr. Booth's article:

"Dr. Evans, the first modern writer on the psychology of cancer, compared cancer patients to clinging vines: once the tendrils have been pulled off the support they are incapable of attaching themselves to a new object. This is not always the case, fortunately, but it is important to realize that *the individualism of cancer patients makes new object relationships particularly difficult.* They are not as flexible and as open to new relationships as, for instance, tuberculosis patients generally are."

"Physicians have reported since ancient times that cancer often follows the loss of an important personal relationship which is experienced as irretrievable. This impression has been validated in recent years by LeShan in clinical and statistical studies. It is significant that it is not an infectious or degenerative process but a localized growth, which follows the loss. Knowing the intense emotional investment of the cancer patient in his original object the tumor impresses as a striking symbolic substitute for what has been lost.

"Unlike the original object, the cancer is firmly entrenched in the body to grow as long as life lasts. Only very powerful outside intervention can remove it. Unconscious introjection of a lost love object has been described originally by Freud as the psychological mechanism of *depression.* In the latter case the patient turns part of his own person into what has been lost, but only in his mind. In cancer, part of the body is transformed into malignancy. Cancer, in other words, is a *somatic form of depression, a sign that something important has been lost.* Unless adequate restitution is made, life will not be supported."

According to Dr. Booth most cancer patients usually conceal psychological situations in which they were previously involved.

"Perhaps the most shocking example of concealment," says Dr. Booth, "occurred in the case of a man who entered psychotherapy on account of a depression. It had begun in an externally very successful period of his professional life. He appeared very trusting and frank, but became worse until, after two years, suddenly symptoms of lung cancer became manifest. Although the diagnosis was made promptly, he delayed the operation until it was too late. He never revealed, even after the operation, what had preceded the organic illness. After two years, however, the only witness of the traumatic incident came to me for a 'confession.' The visitor was a married woman to whom my patient had been devoted for many years. This I had known, but he talked about his involvement always in an ironical manner. Various love affairs and an intense professional life had provided considerable satisfaction until the beginning of the depression. What happened a few days before the first cancer symptoms appeared was a desperate and humiliating attempt to seduce the lady which had been rejected. In the hospital my patient continued to refer to his old friend in the previous ironical manner, but now, because she failed to visit him unlike many more recent acquaintances.

"Many who developed malignancies had given, even to close family members, the impression of leading uncomplicated and happy lives because they had maintained *secrecy regarding a vital involvement.* This specific tendency of cancer victims must be always kept in mind if one wants to help them psychologically. They are likely to be reluctant to talk about 'the heart of the matter.' It requires a very confiding and non-judgmental relationship if one wants to open up about their predicaments. As I have pointed out, they need a close relationship very much, but they are also sensitive to any rejection of their own values and terms.

"You see that it was very logical that the medical profession turned to the clergy for help in their struggle with cancer. This development was due, not so much to a conscious understanding of the religious meaning of the problem, but to the force of the practical situation. The physical situation of the modern cancer patient spells out graphically the predicament of human isolation. The more elaborate and the more accomplished therapeutic techniques have become, the less time physicians and nurses can devote to the moral support of the sick. The latter, all too often, have nobody to whom they can turn except the clergy. In order to meet their crying need, the American Medical Association developed its new program for closer cooperation between physicians and ministers.

"The cancer patient is a person who has been grievously frustrated in some important relationship with the world. The experience has caused the disease which threatens to kill him sooner or later. The disease as such involves a vicious circle: it makes him feel guilty and the guilt feelings often impair his efforts to seek help in good time. If he succeeds in getting proper medical treatment he is given a new lease on life. At this point, his human environment, and particularly his clergyman, are challenged to take advantage of this opportunity.

"I am certain that the minister can *contribute* to physical healings, but only as the indirect result of having helped cancer patients to relate more fully to their fellows and God. More than others they are the victims of the isolation of modern man. This is the reason why their plight has caused the medical profession to turn so earnestly to the clergy for their cooperation. Science can not make man the master of life. We physicians have begun to heed the lesson taught by the spreading of malignant disease. We trust that clergymen will help the cancer patients in their deep need for spiritual reconciliation."

After reading what precedes in this chapter one must realize that anything one can do to change their character, working towards developing a more happy disposition, can reduce the possibility of one getting cancer. We must not overlook the general health factor in making this possible. A sick person generally is more prone to being depressed.

CHAPTER 12

Dr. Elida Evans

BY GOOD FORTUNE there fell into my hands a book called *A Psychological Study of Cancer* (Dodd, Mead and Co.) by Elida Evans, an analyst. The interesting fact about it is that it was published way back in 1926, and that entire book is proof, case by case, that happy people rarely get cancer.

I will give some excerpts from it:

"Every few days a new theory is offered to explain the mystery of cancer, it has become a popular subject. Certainly a great deal of energy has been wasted in following false trails. For many years long and laborious research with large sums of money has been followed in Institutes of Cancer Research, using countless numbers of small animals, such as mice, rats, and guinea pigs for inoculation with most varied and careful detail. Both medical and surgical aspects have been studied, but all the research and experimentation have failed to find a cause or cure.

"The medical profession has been rather reluctant to search for other than physical causes. From ancient habits of thought physicians put everything under the microscope and avoid the mental realm, or, they read one or two books on the subject, attempt psychological work, flounder around, and turn with relief to their prescriptions.

"These newer theories are the result of fifteen years of study, collecting what data I could, during my work with nervous patients whenever their associations brought a reference to cancer, collecting the history of each association as fully as possible.

"I began to find a similarity in their psychological histories, until the cancer patients took the form of a distinct type. The study of one hundred cases is but a drop in the ocean of humanity, but when I began to find parallel cases with the same characteristics, the same habits and conditions, it became interesting."

A Disease of Civilization

"After working for several years with the nervous patients sent to me, and seeing how many ills of the flesh were psychogenic, I expressed an opinion to a physician that cancer might have such a factor. He agreed with me, but added: 'It would not do to say so, it might lead only to further fatal experimentation.' And here lies the difficulty. A medical man hesitates to put full knowledge of any disease into publicity and especially the disease under discussion, fearing it would produce needless and mischievous apprehension of cancer—'cancerophobia.' We know there is heart disease phobia, appendicitis phobia, syphilis phobia, tuberculosis phobia. These phobias are so often found among medical students, probably physicians fear the lay reader would be even more unreasonable.

"About twelve years ago the American Society for the Control of Cancer was started by a small group of physicians in their endeavor to overcome the appalling ignorance existing in regard to this disease, so the public would not hide ostrich-like from its threatening dangers. The only means of overcoming was by education. But alas, the only outcome of their knowledge thus far has been to advise the earliest possible operation, instruction how to avoid chronic irritation and to understand the danger signals. A few faint voices have been lifted that right living would prevent cancer.

"Cancer is a symbol, of something going wrong in the patient's life, a warning to him to take another road.

"We are told by doctors living and practicing in the wilds of Africa and Asia that carcinoma is rarely found among primitive tribes. It is generally conceded to be a disease of civilization.

"Among the opinions given by physicians is that of a German, Dr. F. Cohnheim: 'Cancer is far more common among persons of overweight than among underweights, and by inference among the well-to-do and overnourished than among the less prosperous element.'"

Here is a most astounding statement, made by Dr. Evans in 1926:

"An English writer claims to have found that the real and true cause is lack of vitamins in foods and the toxic poisons which come from indigestion and constipation, and he has written a good-sized volume to explain it with no end of statistics and quotations."

Dr. Evans says that "The soundest opinion of the day believes it (cancer) to be an individual disease, in other words, an excessive and uncontrolled response of the cells of the body to *some type of damage,* (italics mine) either by irritating substance or by inflammation induced by bacteria, or other means."

What he means by "other means" is that the cell can be damaged by psychological factors, which is the whole crux of his book.

Dr. Evans quotes famous psychologist, Dr. Jung as follows:

"A similar effect is produced by the dissociation of the personality, or the disintegration of consciousness as a result of a violent effect of nervous shock, or the dissolution of the personality." These last lines have a direct bearing on our subject of cancer.

"Every extraverted personality thinks, feels and acts in relation to the object, and this condition we observe in the cancer patients and in such direct and noticeable fashion that no one can doubt the patient's dependence upon the object.

"If a person is an intellectual extravert he *thinks,* if a feeling extravert then the subject *'feels himself into'* the object. The latter we find to have been the case with cancer patients, who have put their life energy into a business, an ambition, an ideal or an affection to such an extent they have become part of it.

"Feeling is primarily a process that takes place between the ego and a given content, a process that imparts a definite value to the content in the sense of acceptance or rejection. This 'feeling-into' is a condition we find in the cancer patients, and with such an intensity it results in a state of feeling accompanied by appreciable bodily enervation. They draw their vital needs from the object and are absolutely dependent upon the object for their well-being."

Creative Work

Isn't this reminiscent of the woman in chapter 1, who regularly cleaned a certain church and was discharged by the minister? She had been drawing her vital needs from the church and was absolutely dependent upon it for her well-being. When she was gruffly discharged the thought of it kept growing in her mind until it was all-consuming; at the same time the cancer developed which consumed her body.

"The cancer cell begins in a mysterious way, without order, with instincts perverted. The former, creative, independent life of the patient has stopped, for something depended upon has failed him and this instinct for growth runs wild over the life it seizes.

"In each case where a thorough investigation was possible, we have found there has been a great mental suffering, a total destruction of hope, a tearing asunder of life from life of the patient.

"The one inevitable law of nature is that we must produce results, must accomplish something, otherwise there are nervous troubles of regression to childish actions, such as we find in sweet, placid people, with their fancy work, games and books. We do not know what else we are here for other than to reproduce and *do* something. Even in the static life of the vegetable something is accomplished, seeds are produced."

Dr. Evans evidently believes that if a person is immersed in creative work then some grievous blow that attacks him will not affect him as deeply as a person who has nothing in life to look forward to. Thus he says, "The Linnaean classification of the three kingdoms, 'Stones grow, plants grow and live, animals grow, live and feel,' should include a fourth: 'Human beings grow, live, feel and work,' in either physical or mental labor. Failure of accomplishment, interference with the unfolding ability is disastrous and threatens the extinction of the race. It means for the individual, discouragement, cessation of effort, and moral death, depending upon the freedom with which the energy, the urge of life can act. We are not all born with equal ability, nor of the same quality, for the stock we come from makes a vast difference in us. We are made up of the material our ancestors have given us, and we must really use it to accumulate more material to pass on to our descendants, either in art, science, literature, or in cultivation of the gifts or tendencies we were born with. So far as research has shown, the cancer patient is of healthy stock, but in some way has been interfered with in using the material with which his ancestors have endowed him.

"Unlike the infantilism of the alcoholic, the epileptic, or the tuberculous patient, the cancer patient either has made or has been willing to make a good start, and then has been up against a heart desertion of the beloved object, or a vital separation from the objective aim, but this has not always been apparent to the friends or relatives.

"Men, denied their natural functions either from a frigid wife, or some really legitimate reason, seek satisfaction for existence and pleasure in their food, and cancer of the stomach is most common with them.

"Where there are no children, no marriage, or a most uneven mating, as the fun-loving person with the quiet introvert, the malignant disease appears earlier, and searching through their history we find the same heart-breaking of the objective attachment."

Case Histories

The following are case histories offered as examples by Dr. Evans:

"An instance of this willful, unguided feeling on the part of the cancer patient was found in a woman of 42, unmarried, and a trained nurse. With more than the usual keenness of perception, she understood quite well the whims of her patients, her strong determination served as a prop for them to lean on. She was often praised for her work and invited to the patients' homes to bring some beauty into her life, as an opposite of the hospital atmosphere. 'Beauty,' she said, 'I see no beauty. Human nature is weak and disgusting, with only a surface covering of clothes and smiles.' The house physician heard of her remark, and out of kindness of heart, to relieve such hardness of outlook, talked many times with her. They were in the suburbs of a large city. 'See, are not the birds beautiful? Listen to their songs,' he reasoned with her, 'and the flowers, are not the colors exquisite? Go in the woods and see the majestic beauty of the trees. See the sunlight glistening on the dancing waters of the brook. Listen to the tenderness of nature as the wind whispers among the leaves, and to the tremendous grandeur of its power in the storm.' But no, she could not. This beauty-loving physician felt sad for her, knowing the world must be a hard place for one who saw only the misery of life. Realizing his need of the peace and beauty of nature to balance the opposite of misery and suffering of his patients, he worked on her, hoping to arouse her finer nature.

"At last she came to him. It was the springtime. She told him of a dream she had, in which it was spring, and she was walking through the woods. She heard the birds and felt their musical notes were of a wonderful beauty, but found in her hand a child's whirring rattle and whirled it with all her might. The harsh noise stopped the birds.

"By these thoughts in her sleep she showed she absolutely refused to change herself. Her highly extraverted type could not think it out and acknowledge her need. We learned she had seized the physician who had tried to help her as her objective, and true to type, totally ignored the fact that he was a married man with children. She wanted his personal attention and looked neither to the right nor wrong of her wishes. She began domineering him, his work, telling him of his mistakes, blaming him for his failures, until she became impossible even among the nurses and patients. Later, she had to submit to an amputation of the left breast, and openly declared she had no use for men, women had much more heart. I have found, however, a strong sex urge, a great longing for a normal sexual outlet, even among people of seventy years."

* * *

"While in Switzerland I met a charming woman who told me of her friend's approaching death from cancer. There was the same history of loneliness and separation. The two children had married and moved away, the father and mother were left alone. He was a professor of botany in the university, and was either shut in his study writing and arranging specimens, or hunting through the woods for them. Where could she find an objective attachment for warmth of living? Another case was that of a professional man. Unable to continue his profession from lack of followers, his life was wrenched from its aim. We wondered why, and learned that, of a peculiar nature, he kept his mother in the background to such an extent that when his trouble came of being thrown back on himself he again turned to childish reactions. His wife and children were not his objective aim. His wife was not for companionship, but to keep his house and cook and bear children. His children were to prove to the world that he was a man. He was an extravert as proved by his reading, but he was not a thinker. He read only one side of a question, and evidently read that because education required it. There was no mental food for nourishment in his reading. He filled his library with both sides of a question, and then forgot it. He died from cancer of the stomach. We find in life many a man disappointed in his ambitions or attention, turning to food as a possible means of satisfying that constant craving for something, unknown, or not associated together in his mind. But not so among women. Their cravings are, often quite unknown to them, monogamous and maternal. Do not confuse prostitution with an adult, full-grown craving."

* * *

"Another case of cancer of the stomach was a man, a father, with sons and daughters, and his wife living. He was of decidedly inferior birth and education. But he was a keen business man and made up, he had hoped, by financial success for his lack of social standing. However, his very limited education became more and more apparent as the children grew, and school led on to the question of college. Their father could not spell, and could barely write. His arithmetic was scarcely sufficient for bank accounts, merely addition and subtraction. He indulged his wife and derived all satisfaction in seeing their home the best appointed, his wife and children the best-dressed and riding in the most expensive outfits. While his wife was always proud of her home and her children, and had great respect for her husband's financial ability, she wanted her children educated on her level. Living in a far western city, she longed at times for the opportunities of New York where she was born. The situation became unbearable to her when her husband refused a college education for their sons, fearing it would ruin them for business. She resolved to come East and to live here while the boys were going through preparatory school and college, at least that was an intuitive idea she had, but she did not realize what desertion it would be for her husband nor how dependent he was on his family for his affectionate or emotional outlets, which such a hard-headed man needs to balance up his opposites.

"She entered the three sons in an Eastern school, rented and furnished an apartment in New York, leaving two daughters to keep their father company. But they were up-to-date girls, home did not mean much to them in their free comings and goings. Not being on the same level with their companions, their father suddenly found himself deserted. He attempted to bluff it off and said, 'Oh well, if J. wants to stay and look after the boys in school, I will get a chef and have my own fun.' He did not enjoy his chef, within a month gastric disturbance developed in a cancerous condition. A year and half he lived, most of the time alone, until just at the end when the entire family came. He soon became indifferent about their return, and gave up any interest in them. They declared the chef had caused their father's death. It seemed to me otherwise."

* * *

"Any intelligent person, lay or medical, should realize the importance of keeping up his independent interests, of keeping before him interests which beckon him on, not following from a sense of duty. To do the latter is wearing, and in his unconscious will be found desires and actions to get rid of the duty in most primitive fashion. If a person cannot find a work or interest to fully occupy him, he would better consult a reputable psychologist to dig down and see what is detaining his energy. The interests followed must be such as to fill the follower with relief and keen delight, in the solution, to use up superfluous energy.

"I do not know whether there are statistics of the prevalence of cancer among criminals. I have not met such a case, and they are not a self-sacrificing class. They are not in a position to give of themselves in sacrifice, they are not in a position to give of their best. They have not found themselves and are still seeking. The crimes they commit are overflows from the collective unconscious, indeed they are living in the unconscious only, and have established no individuality. But they are not leaving their creative urge to the collective unconscious, they are actively doing in their consciousness. Instead of being destroyed by it themselves they are destroying others, at one with it.

"Human psychology is like a magic circle, man cannot get out of it, like his skin it surrounds him. It is in him, all through him, it is himself, his life. In order to keep it from falling over to one side we must keep it balanced. We speak of a well-balanced life, but do not know what we must do to keep that balance. It can be expressed in a few words: to watch that the pairs of opposites we possess do not pull us farther on one side than the other. It is only the urge from one opposite that brings the other into force, as the earth is held in place by opposite forces. So do we understand the criminal, as allowing himself to be entirely pulled over to the evil side. Energy must have a balancing between two opposites. There is no life without opposite urge, a flowing in and flowing out of libido. We should learn to think in such terms, and know there can be no energy without opposition.

"The old-fashioned gentle lady, with her embroidery, many servants, and leisurely existence, is passing; the helpless female, depending entirely upon the prim and proper chaperon in youth, upon her husband, home and children in later years, has nearly passed. Athletics, the bicycle and travel have given greater freedom and a broader horizon to both man and woman outwardly, but a large part of mankind are still clinging desperately to whatever they can find as an outlet for their interests and affections. They have not borne the transplanting into a separate existence with the needed vigor. And among them we find the psychogenic phase in their aches and pains, physicians' offices are full of such patients. The victims of the dread disease we are studying have, on the contrary, not been the helpless ones in the beginning. They have started out with full force, and it has not been grief alone which has stopped them. They have had a peculiar kind of sorrow, and a special temperament with which to meet it. They have tried to put their entire selves into their objectives, their stock of libido has rushed out, or tried to, with strong current. But this is an age when the individual must be well rooted to hold his own, he needs several objective aims and attachments. In this mad struggle for a foothold he must seek more than one place to step on to lift himself to higher things.

"We repeatedly find the same history of ambitions and affections thwarted, until it seems that not only does a somatic trauma or irritation result in a malignant growth, but a psychic trauma as well. We have all of us griefs to bear, and deep down in us they remain a painful spot. We try variously to heal over those tender memories by accepting and knowing we must go on with other demands, other ties. But the cancer patient does not seem able to form other ties, perhaps not so much because his conventional bringing up would not allow it, but because it would really be impossible for him to do so from previous conditions. We refuse to be individual, we want someone with us, to share our sorrows, and that cannot be. True, companionship helps tremendously, but we must do our own eating, sleeping, take our own exercise, do our own work. Our muscles will never gain with the exercise another person takes, nor our character develop with the trials other people must endure."

Detached Libido

In his fascinating book, Dr. Evans develops the theory that cancer arises in distinct types of personalities and in response to definable psychological problems. One characteristic that Dr. Evans says he has observed frequently is that the cancer-prone people are one-sided in their interests, intentions, emotions and relations to persons. In other words, in occupation, marriage and love they tend to put all their eggs into one basket. When circumstances, such as the death of a loved one, compel adaptation and change, they are unable to meet the new situation. They cannot find a new job or start a new business because they cannot give up the old one they have lost, and the same unyielding attitude holds for love and marriage.

Dr. Evans says, "We must acknowledge the relentlessness of truth, even if it is against our education, our prejudices, our traditions. Our optimistic friends take it for granted that *good* will be followed by *better.* Man is constantly inclined to forget that what was once good does not remain good eternally. He goes along the old ways that once were good, long after they have become injurious to him. Only through the greatest sacrifice and untold suffering can he rid himself of this delusion, and discern that what was once good is now perhaps grown old and is no longer good. This is so in the little things as in the big. The ways and customs of his childhood, once so sublimely good, he can barely lay aside even when their harmfulness has long since been proved.

"It is as though in the downfall of the objective attachment of the cancer patient, a compact with evil originates with the creative urge of the instincts in the unconscious, from the thoughtlessness of the 'feeling into' extraverted type who are governed absolutely from the feeling side without discrimination. This invasion of evil into a disappointed life signifies a conversion of something previously good into something definitely harmful. This tendency to fall a victim to the one-sidedness of the unconscious in one way or another, is a great and constant danger to all. It is more marked in the cancer patient, from his peculiar individual make-up, so that the one-sided movement of energy breaks out with a compulsion of wild, furious rage, comparable to the savage 'running amok.' The damming up of energy creates a great pressure in the unconscious, which released has irresistible force.

"Without exception, I have found the life of all cancer patients needed broadening, as plainly seen from the blow to their emotions when detached from their objective attachment. Their 'feeling into' the object of their attachment creates an attitude of trustfulness on the part of the patient, while the real qualities of the object (whether he, she, or it), are in no way altered. The 'feeling into' attitude of the patient tries to imbue the object by projection with his own qualities which have no real existence in the object. It is understandable therefore, when the separation of the patient from the object comes, there is no source for the patient to feed his libido, or energy, on. When this life of the patient is not full enough, not satisfactory enough to grow on its own foundation, he gets rid of himself by pouring all his energy (libido) into the object.

"The extravert puts himself into the object to such an extent that he is not entirely reactive to the environmental stimuli, but more so to the objective happenings. If the object of his attachment has sorrow the patient feels it, and so much so that we find the cancer victim neglects his own needs. His body is of no interest to him, its simple elementary requirements which are indispensable to physical well-being are no longer given consideration. The body suffers accordingly, to say nothing of the soul. Although the extravert pays little heed to the good of his soul in not thinking what reactions he is bound to feel, his family or domestic circle notice it with annoyance and dismay. They tell you: 'He is so foolish in taking care of himself, really does nothing he ought for his health, you have to watch him to see if he is well. He ignores his health.' And again: 'She will do nothing for herself, we have to watch her all the time. If she has a cold coming on she will do nothing to stop it, and a cold you know can generally be stopped if taken in time. If not, it becomes seated and has to run a course. We have told her what to do at the first intimation of an infection, at least to tell us. She never says a word.' The loss of equilibrium is perceived only when abnormal bodily sensations are felt with quite strong force. The cancer patient has that peculiar unbending to commands or attempts at persuasion."

Thus Dr. Evans believes that the kind of person who gets cancer is the kind who devotes himself entirely to some other person or cause. He is either unaware of his own individual needs and desires or he ignores them. Society recognizes him or her as a "sweet" person, an especially nice person, a selfless husband, a devoted mother, a person who can work 16 hours a day but never for his own needs—only for those of someone else. When the someone else rejects the love, or grows up to live his own life, or dies, the sorrow is intense and unconquerable and, Dr. Evans thinks, cancer is the result. Interest in life and hope itself are abandoned, and Dr. Evans says:

"When a life gives up hope it tends to become inert, and this tendency we find in the cancer patient before the disease is discovered, but notice that the power in the urge of life has not been exhausted when we do respond to it; the storeroom of energy has not become emptied. It has moved to another level, a lower level, lower in every sense of the word, the level of ignorance, of following blind inclination. Meeting with no restraining force, this ceaseless urge of energy exists in the unconscious with tremendous power when consciousness is listless, hopeless,—(since the opposite of the conscious always exists in the unconscious)—cannot this constant, ceaseless, creative energy run away with itself by producing more living cells than are required to repair waste? And is that not the reason why the cells produced are always the same cells as the affected part requires in healthful metabolism?"

He gives some illustrative case histories:

"A married woman, husband totally deaf, no children. In her earlier married life there was only a moderate income, she practiced strict economy, and her husband, occupied with business, was rarely at home. As his money increased he grew negligent of his wife. A nodule appeared in the breast and an operation restored her to health.

"There came a great shock when the patient's husband told his wife he had invited a woman and her son of eight to visit and to occupy the new guest-house, summers. The woman was about thirty, the husband of our patient was about fifty. Evidently the boy was a son of the husband, as he resembled the father in figure and inherited some peculiar physical marks. Then our patient's husband told her he was going to adopt the woman of thirty as his—their—daughter, it would be so pleasant for them to have a daughter, and the boy could play around. The frequent absences were explained. The adopted daughter became a member of the family, but living in the last guest-house built, and was the constant companion of the adopted father, taking long auto trips of a week or more with him, being introduced as a daughter. And then the wife was left entirely without servants. Her husband said if she could not manage the house any better, the daughter had better take charge. She moved over to the large house, took complete charge, and the wife was considerably isolated. She tried to make a companion of the growing boy. He, however, was forbidden to associate with the wife, and so this energetic woman, cut off from all use of her energy, cursed her fate for being childless. She shut herself away in her suite of rooms, eating there and seldom going out of the house. Soon cancer grew again in the left breast. Her death occurred in less than a year."

* * *

"A young couple came to board in a neighboring farmhouse, a baby boy was born and offered for adoption with good pay. Our patient adopted the boy, giving him the family name. Her libido flowed out to this child, he became the objective aim, and the enlarged income brought comforts. When the child was four years old the payments suddenly stopped. Presumably the child was illegitimate, and the parent who sent the money had died or lost interest. With two children there came still harder times. There was no place to send the adopted boy, and both the patient and her husband, who was a kindly man, had become fond of the handsome, always smiling lad. The problem was solved by sending her own son to live with a well-to-do aunt, with school advantages, and keeping the adopted son. When six years old this boy died, but the strong maternal in her wanted all advantages for her own son, so he was left with the aunt and school. He resembled the father, and it seemed as though he could not replace the attachment she had had for the dead boy. The loneliness, lack of aim, or something to live for, made her listless and always weary, prostrated by the little boy's death it was said. In a few months a lump came in the right breast. A country doctor tried to drive it away with a system of plasters, but it grew rapidly, and in less than two years she died."

Summary

The essence of the work of Dr. Evans was, on the basis of 15 years of clinical practice with nervous patients and study of the cancer problem, the identification of a distinct type of personality that seems to be more prone to develop cancer. "I began to find a similarity in their psychological histories, until the cancer patients took the form of a distinct type."

What he has found was, first, that the individual who gets cancer falls into the psychological type that was called "extraverted" in the classification system of Dr. Jung and that today is called "outerdirected" in the psychological slang of our time. This type of personality is usually considered a desirable one to have. Such people get along well with others, do not appear to have any major psychological problems and find it easy to make other people like them. As Dr. Evans sees them, however, they are people whose way of getting along in life is to see themselves through the eyes of others, to behave as other people expect them to, and to make themselves excessively dependent on other people for approval, happiness and even a sense of being alive. We all know such people who cannot stand to be alone for even an hour or two, who appear to be model parents, husbands or wives because they always do what is expected of them and have no awareness of any contradictory desires they may have, and who generally make every aspect of their lives dependent on the approval and love of others.

"A congenial social life is an enormous help to the extravert, and business interests which bring him in contact with people will bring him greater success. If there are no sidelines to sustain him, no other interests to follow if the large one fails, no other person to turn to in self-preservation, and the strangle-clutch is broken by the one held so tight and close, then trouble comes."

What it comes down to is that Dr. Evans believes

the cancer-prone are those the world regards as "model" citizens, the ones who devote themselves to careers, to worthy causes and to other people, and derive their happiness entirely from the regard of others. A failure in business, loss of an honored position or death of a loved one can leave them utterly without inner resources on which to fall back. They find themselves without interest in living, with nothing to bring them joy or happiness. And it is in this unhappy and depressed state, Dr. Evans says, that cancer develops. "Like a vine torn off from its supports, the cancer patient does not and cannot start a new growth. There is all that length of time, like the length of vine which grew with strong supports while its tendrils clung, and like the old tendrils that cannot unite again to an object. That is a part of life which is past and cannot be lived again, either for the vine or the individual. A vine does not tear itself off from a building, it is a human touch which does it, and so with the cancer patient. It is no self-will of the patient, for his life depends upon the continuity of his relation with the object. It is the inflexibility of his nature which creates another kind of self-will to cling to an idea which in the end destroys him."

And here are some more of the cases with which Dr. Evans goes a long way toward proving his point:

A woman, the second wife, with two stepsons, and a son and daughter of her own. She was the village type of person, living in a small circle of friends, knowing them intimately, enjoying with them the latest bit of news about their neighbors, enjoying especially having her sons bring in the news items they had gathered during the day, and sitting at the table long after the meal was finished to talk over, in an exchange of news, the doings of the small village. She was an incessant talker, words flowed along without effort, but it was difficult for her to get an audience at times. Her husband was an introvert, as silent as she was talkative. The boys had no interest, and the daughter felt her young life was being starved for the social needs of a young girl. So again we find the same old story, the mother full of energy she could not use. Although an extravert, the mother wrote out some of her thoughts she could not express to an audience. At the time of the babyhood of her youngest child, finding no companionship with her husband, she formed an attachment with a neighboring woman. They found a great satisfaction in their intimacy, the neighbor a strong masculine kind of woman, the patient very feminine. While the patient was nursing the baby the neighbor watched and admired the beautiful scene of a nursing mother, calling attention to the whiteness of the perfectly moulded breast. Her regression from the husband was not understood by him, he lived his inner life, running away from disagreeable things, including his wife. He finally hanged himself, we do not know why, excepting that the difference in type from his wife made him even more alone than if unmarried. After the neighbor-woman moved away, our patient was left with no sympathetic understanding. Not the thinking type, she could understand neither the cause of her loneliness, nor how her inability to adapt herself left her alone. When the nodule was found in her breast she had it amputated, but too late. After her husband's death she was left with only the 18-year-old daughter to care for her. This was much too difficult for a young girl with her life unlived; perhaps inheriting or imitating the father type, she was not always sympathetic. But the patient could not change, unable to think out the home situation, and she died with cancer.

* * *

A married man of 52, tall, handsome, very extraverted, prosperous, having large social and business connections. He had an unusually attractive wife, eight children, all well born and grown to adult years in perfection of mental and physical growth. Our patient branched out in business, successful in every undertaking, until he finally brought all his interests and energy into one large enterprise. He was successful in that for many years, his family enjoyed European travel, and evidently expense in living was never considered. Being of the feeling type he did think out the consequences of his impulsive acts. He was surrounded with men whom, in his kindness and generosity, he had advanced to very responsible positions. His unfailing large heart could not understand the meanness and smallness of human nature, the opposite type to himself, and while the pull from his large ego was towards generosity, in his employees it was from the sordid side. He went on thus until at the very brink of destruction, when he found his most trusted men were combining against him to get him out of the presidency of the company he had founded with his capital and experience. His board of trustees elected another man in his place, his power became nil, and the stock, which had been largely his own, he had to use for the expenses and growing demands from the increased needs of his large family. The salary of his official position had been large, and not having the kind of mind that can think and reason from the subjective side, he did not realize the insecurity of his position until too late. He suddenly found himself a ruined man. He went home to his wife, who like him was of a buoyant nature, very extraverted, and they saw no way out of their dilemma. He sold more stock, and lived from the frequent sales until his death from cancer of the bladder.

* * *

A man of 44 years, married, two children, a self-made man of keen business ability. He had worked since childhood, beginning at six years to support himself, so he had had very little education. But gay and lively, when 22 he had attracted a girl of 18 into a violent love affair. She came from an upper social class and was forbidden any acquaintance with the patient. But he with his wild life of perfect freedom, never having had any restraint or opposition to his wishes, proposed they elope, and they did so. He was an untamed man of lower type, she an artistic, refined woman. It was remarkable that he could satisfy her. He probably recognized her superiority and worshiped her for it, giving her all the credit in the shops she needed to supply their home, the children and herself. Early in their married life he found her extravagant in his opinion, so allowed her credit in any shop in the town but very little cash in hand. He knew well how hard it was to earn money, while she had no idea of its value. He thought she did not need money with a limousine and unlimited credit, but she did, and it must have been torture with her refined tastes never to be able to gratify them in matters of dress and home furnishing, as a woman enjoys so much picking odd and dainty trifles.

As her children grew old enough for discipline and to begin school, his ideas and methods were a great trial to her. He wanted them to begin work at the earliest possible age and to go to night school. His wife was horrified, she had looked forward to college for the boys, as he was no help in training them, having had practically no training himself. A few years in public school was enough for them, he insisted, and opposed education so strongly it became a taboo subject. If he could not manage his own children, he said, he would have no more, and he moved to a distant part of the house. His wife became crippled with neuritis, spent years in a sanitarium, where she suffered less, but always mourned for her children, her home, and longed for her husband. He lived on in the home with servants they had had for years, avoiding all women, and the children had a lonely time. They began to turn away from their father, asked for their mother, and he found himself without their affection, his wife away, and a great sense of loneliness seized him. He declared man could not live without the love of wife or children, but refused to change his ideas of education and could not understand why he was left alone and unloved. He had put all his pride, affection and hope in the refined wife as the feeling-extravert type. When she failed him he turned to his children. They openly called him "an old skinflint" and avoided him. He asked, "Why is it that I am now left alone when I need my family so much? It makes me sick to think how I have slaved for them, and now find myself deserted." True to the cancer type, he would not bend from his wishes and ideas, could not see how one-sided he was and that all the world could not live by his rigid model.

His neighbors thought his constantly being tired and his loss of appetite were due to his loneliness. It was found, however, that he had developed cancer in the intestinal tract. He refused to have his wife told of it until the last, as she was still crippled from neuritis in a distant sanitarium.

The last week of his life she was brought home. He was too ill and weak from the suffering and starvation of the cancer growth to talk of the past. She recovered very rapidly, and walked in a few days. After his death she stayed home with only occasional light attacks of neuritis. One year later a nodule was found in the breast. An immediate radical operation prevented further growth. After several years she is well and active, with abundant outlet for her energy in a home life with her sons and their companions.

* * *

A widow of uncertain age, over 40. Her husband had died when she was 27 leaving her with a daughter of eight years.

When she was 19 her little daughter was born. She was still living with her parents. Eight years later her husband died. As he had not been the love of her young life she easily turned her objective aim to the parents and baby girl whose growing demands of clothes and schools occupied the mother. The child, however, was too full of her own individuality to be a constant companion to her mother, and later she married. A sisterly relation existed between the mother and daughter. Then came financial reverses with the death of the daughter's husband. She was obliged to become self-supporting, to support her mother and herself, but did not tell her mother of their reverses. The mother became one with her daughter, "feeling-into," throwing all her individuality in her daughter and with no aim of her own. This made an impossible situation for the daughter. In self-defense she was obliged to put the mother out of her thoughts to keep from being utterly exhausted, and to have any freedom of action. It necessitated frequent absences from home to rest and to get herself free for collecting more energy, which left the mother without any support, like the vine torn from its clinging. Her daughter seemed very hard-hearted to the mother, who refused to see that the daughter needed any life of her own, but was judged as being "just like her father, strong-willed." But really it was the mother who was strong-willed, who would not busy herself in any occupation during her daughter's daily absence at an office where she worked. The mother constantly blamed the daughter, finally turned against her and preferred to live away with more congenial people, she said, and then attempted suicide.

After recovering from that, her failing strength showed an internal cancer had started in an inoperable place, the bladder, which caused her death.

* * *

A man of 50, married, seven children, three of them married, developed an internal cancer and died. As we look over his history we note the same distressing facts. As a youth, his disposition was gay, happy and sunny. He was fond of all social doings and was the life of every dinner or gathering. His light was never hidden under a bushel, laughter and good cheer surrounded him. His flow of vocabulary was a gift, and if the English language failed to express his meaning he coined endless words, to the displeasure of his family.

When 20 years of age he finished school and entered an importing firm of which he later became a member. This highly extraverted young man married a girl deeply introverted and just his opposite. She was quiet, very attractive, dark-haired, had a winning smile showing flashing white teeth, but was shy, avoiding people and really most unsuitable for such a man. He was demonstrative, constantly wanting to embrace her and show his affection, which was annoying to her. He had a habit which I have noticed in many cancer patients, and that is, using baby talk. The rapidly arriving babies gave his wife an excellent excuse for a quiet home life, while the father played and romped with the children as though of their age.

In his firm he became very intimate with his two partners, and being of the feeling-extraverted type his relations with them became brotherly. Their business was a success financially. I do not know if the very close friendship which our patient felt for his partners was mutual. After quite a number of years, business troubles came to him. His two partners died within a short time of each other, and their families wanted their share of the firm's money. Our patient, true to his type, feeling-extravert, unable to think it out and realize he would not have capital enough left to carry on such a large business, immediately began to pay the widows their share. Of course he failed in a few years. The mortgage on his home, a large place in the suburbs, was foreclosed. His wife was very sympathetic, we hope, but she did not say anything to comfort him. She accepted the reverses, and the children, then grown, the youngest 16 years, tried to show their affection for the father by being more patient with his baby talk.

Like the mother, the four unmarried children were introverts. They, with their mother, were amazed to find the father as cheerful and optimistic as ever. A friend had bought the house and rented it to our patient for a nominal amount, so the home was kept. A married son brought his wife and baby to the parental home, and with a few young men of business connections boarding in the house, a sufficient income was gathered for living expenses. As troubles increased the patient's cheerfulness increased, laughter, jokes, teasing his family with exaggerated baby talk and increased hugging and kissing of wife and three unmarried daughters, which affected them as it naturally would introverted types. Their inflowing libido could not rush out to him when he was so sadly in need of it to compensate for his forced cheerfulness. The whole situation began to change. The mother found it most difficult at times to endure her husband's cheerfulness in the presence of strangers, she left the family board and ate always in her room. The four children blamed their father for the mother's withdrawal from the family circle, they frowned on him, said cutting things. The son remarked, "Dad is so damned cheerful it is too much for me," and frequently left the table.

Then began the father's regression. Practically cast off by his family, his libido sought satisfaction in his food. Always a *bon vivant,* he now began to eat enormously. In a year the fatal disease was discovered. He had grown very stout, but his cheerfulness left him. It was difficult to keep up his small business interests and he finally gave up going to his office. He tried to cling to food for satisfaction, gradually his appetite failed but he "wished someone would fix up something nice and dainty." His artistic wife and unmarried children did not do so, his baby talk increased in proportion and his family turned away from him. "All that's left to feed on now is cold shoulder, not of lamb, but the family shoulder." It was almost his last joke. When the physician discovered the presence of carcinoma, the family were horrified. "I am cut off in my prime," he said, "I am starved and frozen and knocked up." His family were unable to show their love for him and wept in private, avoiding him to hide their red eyes, thinking it would spare him, while he still craved the affection denied so many years. His wife rarely went into his room. "Lie down beside me, put your face against mine, hold my hand, kiss me," he asked his wife. But she ran away to her room instead. "If Benny's and Dan's (his former partners') children had come into the firm when they were still young they would have learned the business and it would have been saved. But Mary and Sarah (the partners' wives) never had any heart, so they are alive and well. I tried and tried to show those boys how they could take up the old firm and make it a success. They laughed at me. It was the last straw, cold shoulder at home and in the office starves a man. I give it up, I don't care." His life of usefulness so suddenly stopped was not satisfied. We see the regression, the renunciation of effort, his unwillingness to change, to adapt himself to another business, and rushing out in true feeling-extravert type to his family, partners' family and his friends, until they had to avoid him. As he abandoned all effort he left the opposite sex and sought boys and men for companionship. His death occurred in less than a year from the discovery of the malignant growth.

CHAPTER 13

Some Comments by Doctors

"Let me speak to you regarding the things of which you must most beware. To get angry and shout at times pleases me, for this will keep up your natural heat; but what displeases me is your being grieved and taking all matters to heart. For it is this, as the whole of physic teaches, which destroys our body more than any other cause."

The physician who wrote thus to his patient was Maestro Loranze Sassoli, and he inscribed this letter in the year 1402. He was revealing a common medical notion of the times that cancer, specifically, was related to one's temperament. Galen, the father of modern medicine, who lived in the second century A.D., believed that melancholic women were more prone to cancer than those whom we today would call happy-go-lucky.

By the 18th century European physicians were noting in their medical articles that a severe emotional shock (usually the death of a loved one) contributed to a large extent to the onset and development of cancer. Physicians of that time had available none of the tests which modern researchers use to discover facts about personality and personality difficulties. So they could do nothing but record their observations about personality and cancer.

Here are some of the notes they made:

1822—Nunn described a woman who died of breast cancer shortly after the death of her husband.

1846—Walshe wrote in part as follows: "Much has been written on the influence of mental misery and habitual gloominess of temper on the deposition of carcinomatous (cancerous) matter. If systematic writers can be credited, these constitute the most powerful cause of the disease; and Lobstein, assuming the fact as established, exercised his ingenuity in tracing the connection of the cause and effect: moral emotions produce defective innervation, this perversion of nutrition which in turn caused the formation of carcinoma (cancer) . . . I have myself met with cases in which this connection appeared so clear that I decided questioning its reality would have seemed a struggle against reason."

On the basis of this conviction Walshe advised patients with a family background of cancer to select their professions with great care. Avoid those which entail constant care and anxiety, he cautioned. Clearly, he believed that an inherited tendency to cancer plus a long-term period of psychological stress might result in cancer.

1885—Willard Parker, an American, studied 97 cases of breast cancer and reported that grief is undoubtedly associated with the disease. Cancer patients are not people who have been noted for cheerfulness before the disease struck them. Another physician, Cutter, remarked that mental depression is too often an element in cancer to be overlooked. He believed, furthermore that the disease could be cured by diet and by stimulating the patient's will to live.

An English physician reports, "Great mental stress has been assigned as influential in hastening the development of cancer. Another said that cancer of the breast and uterus follow immediately upon depressing emotion, too often to be mere chance.

By 1921 Willy Meyer, who introduced radium therapy for cancer into America, wrote that he believed that cancer is often the result of social and emotional stress because of changes in the body produced by such stress —in other words, changes in the actual chemistry of the body necessitated by its reaction to severe stress.

As psychoanalysis became popular, as the ideas of Freud and Jung received wider acceptance, we find analysts stating that cancer is an "acting out of deep frustrations" by the body. Here are some other more modern viewpoints:

Physical Habits Influence Mental Condition

Hoffman, writing in 1915, "From dietary disorders to nervous disorders is but a step. The two are frequently interrelated and cause and effect are often hopelessly confused . . . This naturally brings me to the question of the interrelationship of cancer and worry, or the mental attitude of the patient toward the development, spread and curability of the disease." Another researcher, Foque, in 1931 spoke of the "role of sad emotions as activating and secondary causes in the activation of human cancers." His theory, important and well-conceived, we believe, was that stress or emotion affects the nervous system which in turn affects the body's metabolism, which acts on the glands in such a way as to make individual cells susceptible to the effects of a cancer-causing substance. He spoke of his patients thus, ". . . you can see in the patients prolonged and silent sorrow without the release of sobs and tears."

He and many other modern writers believed that the death of a child, a spouse or another loved one, plays an important part in the chain of events that result in cancer.

As statistical methods were developed for studying such theories, it was found that indeed this appeared to be the case. In different marital conditions among women it might be presumed, therefore, that there would be the largest incidence of cancer among widows, the next largest incidence of cancer among those who had been divorced or separated, less among those who were legally married whether or not much remained of a happy relationship, and least cancer among single women. A survey of cancer statistics in 1956 showed that this was the case, where there were adequate statistics to work with. Other statistical studies seemed to show similar trends. Invariably widows in all age groups had a higher cancer mortality than happily married or single women.

Psychiatrists delved deeper and found that apparently there was a relationship between incidence of cancer and unhappy relationship between other members of the family, especially, so it seems, an unresolved conflict with the mother of the family. Extensive studies have been done showing that there is apparently a very definite connection between certain kinds of personality and cancer incidence. Time and again the "cancer personality" is described as a person who has a defensive attitude toward society, more anxieties than normal and less ability to reduce tension by some outward manifestation. That is, the person who broods silently rather than shouting when he is angry; the person who grieves and harbors silent fears and grudges, who cannot "work off" a feeling of depression, anger or frustration with exercise, singing, hard manual labor, or loud talking.

Then, too, there seemed to be a certain undoubted relationship between emotions and the state of a patient who had finally succumbed to cancer. We are told by Trunnell in a paper read at a cancer symposium in 1956 that almost without exception the cancer patient reacts with certain definite emotional and physical changes to the degree of illness or the deaths of patients around him. The need for narcotics varies, there are chemical changes in the urine and so forth.

In *Cancer and Personality: A Critical Review* by Lawrence LeShan, published in the January, 1959 issue of the *Journal of the National Cancer Institute,* the author tells us that such investigations as he reports in this article (which we have covered briefly above) do not give us a cure for cancer. Easing the emotional strains of the patient will not necessarily halt the disease. "One does not put out a forest fire by extinguishing the match that started it," he says. "It is nevertheless true that it may be necessary, after putting out the fire, with other means, (surgery, radiation or chemotherapy) to extinguish the match in order to prevent a new fire."

We would add—isn't it a better idea to warn against match-lighting and so prevent the forest fires from ever starting in the first place?

Dr. LeShan's conclusions—and we think they are important for all health seekers to know—are: that there seems to be a certain relation between some emotional states of mind, some kinds of personality and cancer. The loss of a loved one seems to be one of the most common starting points for cancer. There also seems to be some relationship between the kind of personality one has and the time newly-discovered cancer results in death. And there seems to be some connection, little understood, between the kind of personality and the location of cancer.

What We Can Learn from This Research

We know that diet and way of life have a great deal to do with one's adjustment to life and its inevitable sorrows and stresses. This is obvious from the fact that deficiencies in certain essential nutriments can produce within a short time depression, nervousness, anxiety, even in individuals who had previously been happy, strong and self-reliant. Depriving test volunteers of the B vitamins alone brings about results of this kind.

We know, too, that stress situations are wasteful of vitamins and minerals. Loss of a loved one is perhaps the most acute stress any of us is subjected to. There is no doubt that all the body changes that accompany such a shock use up one's supply of food elements. For those who do not immediately replace them, it seems only reasonable that a serious disease like cancer might get a strong foothold at such a time when all resistance is low.

Then, too, it seems obvious that prolonged stress over years of quarreling with one's family or associates or resenting the things they do, without showing open hostility, would be bound to take a serious toll in one's physical makeup, once again making one more susceptible to the onset of a disease.

On the other hand doesn't it seem possible, too, that it is the ill, badly nourished people who are the ones most likely to have emotional difficulties? We all know families in which some are happy, easy to get along with and well adjusted to their jobs and their associates, while others in the same family are irritable, "difficult," nervous, depressed. Doesn't it seem that the same set of prenatal conditions, childhood and adolescence habits and diet which produced the unhappy personality may also, later on, produce the cancer?

Sir Heneage Ogilvie said, "The instances where the first recognizable onset of cancer has followed almost immediately on some disaster, a bereavement, the break-up of a relationship, a financial crisis, or an accident, are so numerous that they suggest that some controlling force that has hitherto kept this outbreak of cell communism in check has been removed."

While the thinking about the relationship between emotions and cancer remains in its present stimulating but unresolved state, it seems to us that the best idea is to do everything you can to avoid being the kind of person who seems to be most susceptible to cancer—depressed, silent, worrying, anxious, resentful or "all wrapped up in yourself."

Aside from a definite conscious effort to turn one's thoughts in a happier direction, there is the necessity to do everything possible to create a body so radiantly healthy that happiness is unavoidable.

CHAPTER 14

A Recent Study

UP TO NOW, we have dealt with fairly esoteric material in that we have investigated the roots of the knowledge of a relationship between cancer and emotional states in early writings on the subject. It would be wrong to believe, however, that modern science is entirely ignoring this intriguing question. Granting that the major efforts of research workers are devoted to such projects as testing hundreds of poisons to try to find one that will be more poisonous to malignant tissue than to healthy, nevertheless there are those who recognize the probable importance of this field of research. It is from such as these, striking out into radically new paths, that we hope for ultimately significant results that will help in the prevention of cancer.

Once such daring research man is Lawrence LeShan of the Institute of Applied Biology in New York City.

For the past 14 years Dr. LeShan has been studying what he calls the "emotional life histories" of adult cancer patients, looking for a common pattern that might be linked to the incidence of cancer. In April of 1965, when his study had been going on for 12 years, he was able to report on preliminary results to a conference on psychophysiological aspects of cancer held by the New York Academy of Sciences. At that time Dr. LeShan reported on 450 patients, all of whom had given extensive written personal histories on a well-designed test, and 150 of whom had been interviewed for an average of four hours each. Studying these histories, Dr. LeShan was able to find a remarkable similarity forming what he called a pattern of development and relationships that he found in 72 per cent of the cancer patients, while the same pattern was found in only 10 per cent of the non-cancerous controls that he used. (Although he did not mention the possibility, it is not unlikely that cancer later developed or will develop in the 10 per cent of the controls who showed the same type of emotional pattern as that which was found dominant in cancer patients.)

Emotional Damage in Childhood

The first common element that Dr. LeShan stated as being dominant in emotional histories of cancer patients was that at some time during the first seven years of life, some kind of severe emotional experience damaged the ability of the child to relate to other people and to life itself. This could have been and often was a death in the family, such as the loss of one parent or of a brother or sister. In some cases it was simply the birth of a younger brother or sister and the loss of a great deal of parental attention and love which was shifted to the newborn. Whatever the specific cause, the child experienced a not uncommon reaction. Having loved someone fully and without qualification, the child experienced a deep pain and sense of loss at being deprived of that love, and came to the conclusion emotionally that it was safer not to love and not to risk the consequent pain of loss of the loved one.

This is a fairly common type of psychological development, leading in many children to an inner sense of guilt and a conviction of unworthiness to enjoy the love of others. Such children very quickly lose all conscious knowledge of why they have detached themselves emotionally from the world around them and only feel that it is because of something missing in themselves, some lack of capacity for life, that they are not able to love people or enjoy living as others do.

Such a psychological deficiency rarely has any obvious signs. The child seems to be fairly well adjusted to the world around him. He does what he is supposed to do, he goes to school, he learns his lessons, he plays games with other children, and it is only by his lack of enthusiasm, perhaps by the inability to laugh, that an occasional perceptive adult may recognize there is something wrong. To most he seems perfectly normal, perhaps even better than others because he will tend to be unaggressive, having little that he really wants. He may also be very helpful to others, feeling more able to relate to the sick, the impoverished or the somehow enfeebled who by their very weakness represent less of a threat.

The net result in the young adult is frequently what is considered a "saintly" personality.

As we have seen before, this type of early personality development leads in turn to an utter devotion poured into a very narrow channel—a business, a husband or wife, perhaps a child. Here is Dr. LeShan's description of the situation:

"Some time in his development, usually in our cases in late adolescence or early adulthood, a situation arose that offered an opportunity for relating to others; a perceived chance to end the deep loneliness he felt. This possibility seemed somehow 'safe.' Over a period of time, a period of slow and cautious experimentation, he began to pour his energies into this channel. The feelings of isolation and 'lostness,' the deep loneliness were greatly, but never completely, eased by this relationship. A tremendous amount of psychic and usually physical energy was poured into it. The cathexis (fixation of the libido or love drive onto an object) gave a meaning to life. For a period ranging from one year to over forty, they had a meaningful existence and a channel into which to pour their energy.

"Sometimes it was a job with a role for which they seemed particularly well adapted and which they enjoyed. Sometimes, as a spouse, a parent, or both, they found a way of life that brought them closer to satisfaction and relatedness than they had ever dreamed was possible. They still found it difficult to express or defend their own wishes, but in the interest of their group or of the relationship, they could act very strongly.

"For a shorter or longer period, life continued on this plane. Then the blow fell. Circumstances brought an end to the relationship; their role was lost. Job retirement was forced on them, a spouse died, children grew up, became independent or no longer needed them. The immediate reaction varies. Some made desperate efforts to find substitute relationships. They tried to obtain new jobs, to make new friends, to find a new group, only to fail. Others were crushed by the blow. From a superficial view, all continued to 'adjust.' They continued to function and went about their daily business, but there was no more meaning and hope to their lives. Nothing gave them real satisfaction. It seemed to them as though the thing they had expected and feared all their lives—utter isolation and rejection—was now their eternal doom. The only way out was to cease existing. 'Half in love with easeful death I cry' seemed to express their feelings. Although they feared death, they did not want to live.

"The early fantasy of something being basically wrong with them, something that made them unacceptable to others, returned in full force. Their energy level declined, because now there was no meaningful channel for its expression, and the decline was soon felt. The color and zest went out of life. *At some time from six months to 8 years after the crucial cathexis was lost, the first symptoms of cancer appeared in the cases we observed.*"

Dominated by Despair

Doctor LeShan found this same basic pattern repeated in 72 per cent of the 450 cancer cases whose emotional history he had painfully secured. What he considers the key factor is the ultimate quality of despair that dominates the person's life. And he defines it as hopelessness about ever achieving any real enjoyment or a real sense of meaning in life. Although the person tries and keeps on trying to establish meaningful relationships, it is always an inner conviction that he is going to fail which in itself leads to failure.

One patient, when interviewed, said, "I go on and I'm very efficient and I function very adequately, but this has nothing to do with the real me. Inside, none of this matters."

As a second described it, "It's as if all my life I've been climbing a very steep mountain. It's very hard work. Every now and then there are ledges I can rest on for a little bit and maybe even enjoy myself a little, but I've got to keep climbing, and the mountain has no top."

A third described his life as being like a house with no insulation and with cracks in the walls. "The more heat you put in, the more heat leaks out. You can never get it warm."

And this type of personality, LeShan found, is overwhelmingly the type that contracts cancer. He carried his study further, however, examining his own and other statistics, particularly a study of the families of 200 breast cancer patients that was made in Copenhagen. This statistical study led LeShan to other significant conclusions. He found a statistical relationship, for example, between marital status and the incidence of cancer. The highest cancer rate was found among those who are widowed with the next highest rate among the divorced. The lowest rate is among single people, with the married in between. Reference to the census vital statistics for both the United States and the British Isles gave complete support to this thesis.

Finally LeShan asks the following significant question:

"Can psychological status of a patient affect the development of his tumor? If we accept a correlation between certain psychic states and neoplastic disease, what happens if the psychic states are modified? It is the author's strong *impression* that the psychotherapy considerably slowed the development of the neoplasm, but no definitive proof can be given at the present time."

Regrettably, Dr. LeShan is in no sense a nutritionist. It apparently has never occurred to him to experiment with such elements as the vitamin- and enzyme-rich Gerson diets that significantly retarded and in some cases cured cases of cancer, or the large, therapeutic quantities of vitamin B and enzyme-rich desiccated liver and brewer's yeast that have been found in other experiments to act as a preventive of the development of cancer. Though we do not say it is so, it is at least possible that part of the effectiveness of these nutrients in combatting cancer may lie in their ability to improve the health of the nervous system and in this way improve and alter the emotional state.

There can be little doubt that there is a complicated and subtle interrelationship between the condition of health of the nerves and the way the mind operates. Which is the chicken and which the egg in the genesis of cancer is a question that no one has ever attempted to answer as yet.

CHAPTER 15

Isolation and Hodgkin's Disease

HODGKIN'S DISEASE, while generally considered a form of cancer, is quite different from any other type of cancer. It is a disease specifically of the lymph glands, including the spleen. And rather than showing tissue cells that are different in character and appearance and form a tumorous mass, the wild proliferation of Hodgkin's disease comes from the uncontrolled overproduction of lymph, which is accompanied by simple swelling of the lymph glands. Since it is a unique form of cancer, the question naturally arises in our study of whether there may be unique personality characteristics that would lead to Hodgkin's disease rather than another form of cancer.

Only one scientific study has been made of this particular question, so far as we can find. It was done by

Lawrence LeShan, of the Institute of Applied Biology in New York, a pioneer and leader in the investigation of the possible relationship between personality and the development of cancer. Published in *Psychological Reports* (Vol. 3, 1957) Dr. LeShan's paper was titled "A Psychosomatic Hypothesis Concerning the Etiology of Hodgkin's Disease."

Most interestingly, his paper opens with the same idea for which we were seeking corroboration or refutation. He states that he was impressed by certain personality characteristics of patients with Hodgkin's disease that distinguish them from those with other forms of cancer. A unique form of cancer occurring to people with a unique type of personality? If so the very fact would go a long way toward proving that personality and the incidence of cancer are indeed related.

Unhappy Childhood

Dr. LeShan made his study by taking 17 consecutive admissions for Hodgkin's disease at the Institute of Applied Biology and adding to them 3 more from a city hospital to fill out the group of 20. There were 9 women ranging in age from 27 to 44 and 11 men, 23 to 53 years of age. The median age for women was 32, while for men it was 26, demonstrating one of the unusual aspects of Hodgkin's disease. It occurs most often in people who are far younger than any other kind of cancer patients.

These Hodgkin's disease patients were compared with three control groups, one made up of 100 people who had been found free of cancer and all other diseases in a screening program, one made up of 35 patients with other forms of cancer who had been equated to the study group for age and social class, and one made up of 200 unselected patients with a wide variety of cancers. Personal histories were taken for all of them and followed up with clinical interviews.

Dr. LeShan says that "This investigation into the life history pattern of patients with Hodgkin's disease revealed a sequence of events which appears more consistently in these patients than in our control groups. This sequence appears to antedate the first-noticed symptoms of the disease by many years, and may have important implications for the pathogenesis and etiology of this process.

"There seem to be three phases in this pattern. The first phase consists of a childhood and adolescence marked by strong feelings of unworthiness and much psychological stress. During this period, the individual appeared to function normally but never related himself to others with any great intensity. Early psychological trauma made the establishment of intense relationships difficult. There was a rich fantasy life and frequently much emotional investment in ideas, but the level of outwardly expressed emotion and of physical activity was normal or slightly below normal.

"During late adolescence or early adulthood, the second psychological phase started. This was marked by the discovery of a peer group with similar goals and orientations. This group provided a focus for the individual's relationship needs. After a period of cautious testing, he felt accepted. The goals and orientations of this group merged with his own and the two became largely identical. Into the activities of the group he poured a tremendous amount of energy. His level of outwardly expressed emotion and physical activity increased very markedly to a degree that was far above normal. His need for sleep was much less than before. He seemed never to tire, always to have energy enough to carry tremendous loads. As long as the relationship with this group was maintained, the high level of energy and physical activity remained constant."

What Dr. LeShan is presenting here is a type of personality development that is quite different from the kind we have previously found related to other types of cancer. The childhood is as unhappy in as profoundly basic a way, but whereas the earlier types we had studied simply repressed their own personality tendencies and became dutiful, obedient and seemingly model children who were not aware of their own unhappiness, the Hodgkin's disease type in Dr. LeShan's evaluation was very much aware of unhappiness as a child. It is pointed out that there was much psychological stress and the child came to feel unworthy. He felt that others would not accept him, presumably as his family did not accept him, because he was not as good, clever, obedient or whatever as other children.

This period of intense unhappiness as a child seems to have been followed by relationship to a group rather than an individual. In our studies of other types of cancer patients, we found a tendency to "fall in love" or in some way build the entire world around one small object—a husband, a child, a job. The Hodgkin's disease patient, on the other hand, is the type that in this creative period focuses less on an individual than on a group, rejoicing in the social aspects of acceptance and devoting himself entirely to the welfare of the social group.

"The third phase of this pattern began with the loss of the relationship to this group for reasons beyond the individual's control, such as graduation from school and induction into the armed services. He now felt isolated and alone, and in spite of the existence of many objective interpersonal relationships, a strong feeling of anomie (being different from the others) was present. For reasons related to his early development, attempts to establish relationships with other groups failed. After a period of intensive attempts either to re-establish the original group or to find a new one, the person abandoned hope and began to despair of being able to find real satisfaction in life. At this time the level of outwardly expressed emotion, physical activity, and available energy dropped off from the very high level of phase two. He now tired more easily, could carry less of a load, and began again as in phase one, to operate at normal or slightly below normal levels of activity and energy. In 18 out of 20 of the cases we studied with the projective test and intensive psychotherapy, the first symptoms of Hodgkin's disease appeared within six months to 8 years after the establishment of phase three."

Superior Intelligence

This describes another strikingly different characteristic consisting of the early abandonment of hope and the experience of despair. Another striking characteristic described by Dr. LeShan is that "all the Hodgkin's patients studied were people of superior intellectual endowment." And he points out that their abilities and high energy potential were blocked off by their isolation, depriving them of channels of expression.

In the balance of his paper, Dr. LeShan speculates on the method of development of the lymph system that could be stimulated by the emotional development into the eventual occurrence of Hodgkin's disease. The material is purely speculative and we can see no point in reproducing it here. What we feel is most important and what we believe Dr. LeShan has gone a long way toward establishing is the definition of a specific type of unhappy personality development that can and sometimes does lead to Hodgkin's disease.

Here are some case histories he offers to illustrate the pattern more concretely:

CASE I.—A 35-year-old male. As a child he had felt awkward and out of place on the family farm. His brothers enjoyed farming and were closer to the parents; his own interests lay in music and were strongly discouraged by the entire family. He recalls frequent childhood predictions that he would never be of any use to anyone and would never be able to earn a living. He felt clumsy, bound to fail. The family's estimate of him was accepted. He had no close friends and felt alone. Telling him that "You've gotta get off the farm, you'll never be any good here," the family sent him to business college in the hope that "I could at least earn my own living." As a member of the choir in college, he came into his own. As it became known that he had a fine voice, he began to receive requests to sing at parties, dances, etc. He found himself popular and began to enjoy this. In his second year at college, he was singing nearly every evening in the week. Between school, music practice, and singing engagements at night he had little time for sleep, but yet never seemed to become tired. For the first time he felt accepted and wanted by others. The choir was his particular joy and he devoted a great deal of time to it.

At graduation he was encouraged to go to Hollywood to sing professionally. He made an attempt to break into the movies or to join a band, but his efforts were not successful. For six years he worked in clothing stores, in department stores and similar jobs, making the rounds of the studios and using what money he could earn to take singing lessons. The only singing jobs he could find were on Sunday mornings in a church choir, but his musical and religious interests were regarded with suspicion. In spite of this rejection, he intensified his interests. He felt more hopeless and depressed as the years went on. He became tired more easily and found himself less active. Six years after college graduation, the first signs of Hodgkin's disease were observed.

Case II.—A 23-year-old male. When he was 5 years old, his father died. At the same time his mother was pregnant. He felt rejected and alone. He felt somehow responsible for the father's death and for the economic pressure on the family. He had few friends in childhood and turned more and more to interests in science. In high school he found others with similar interests and science clubs, and by his junior year was a fully accepted member of a group of students who experimented and worked together, and spent a great deal of time with scientific hobbies. He decided to become an engineer and greatly enjoyed studying and training himself in relevant areas. His hobbies included photography, astronomy, gun smithing, ornithology, and nature studies, which indicated the intensity of his feelings about science. He and his friends invested much emotion, time, and energy in these fields. Somehow there seemed to be time for all of them, as well as for his studies and after-school jobs.

Upon graduation, he felt that he had to help support his mother, since she had worked so hard to send him to school. The plans to become an engineer were reluctantly abandoned and he took a job as a truck driver, which paid him over $70.00 a week. He tried very hard to keep up his interests but was unable to maintain contacts with those he had known in high school, since most of the other members of the in-group went to college and since his hours were long and irregular. He pursued his interests alone but his energy began to flag and he became too tired after his work was finished. Life seemed less rewarding as time went on. Even the fact that he was bringing home money (and thereby easing some of his guilt feelings) brought him no feelings of reward. He was not accepted by his fellow truck drivers which hurt him. Four years after graduation, the first symptoms of Hodgkin's disease were noted.

Case III.—A 32-year-old female. An intellectually driven mother, a submissive and dominated father, and a sister two years younger who was "the beauty," were factors which contributed to this woman's childhood feelings of being rejected and unloved. Her attempts to get love from her mother seemed to her to result only in anger, as they interfered with the mother's social and political interests. The father who had a strongly puritanical background, regarded any physical contact with the daughter as repugnant. She felt unable to compete with the sister in attractiveness. Her one interest was music. She enjoyed her piano lessons and showed unusual talent. In the midst of the extensive social life her family carried on, she preferred to go to her room alone to practice or to read biographies of great musicians.

She left home for college, but her first year there was unhappy and lonely. She did poorly in her studies, had no friends except her music teacher, and as final exams approached, became tense and terrified. The evening before the first exam, she slipped on the sidewalk and badly fractured her shoulder.

Instead of returning to college, she persuaded her family (with the help of her mother's psychotherapist) to let her go to a large city and study piano. She took an apartment with two other girls who were studying art or music and the three became very close. They worked hard at their studying and practicing, and spent long hours talking and exploring the city. "I felt as if new doors were opening to me every day." She learned a great deal about art and music, and "it was a wonderful year. I still feel nostalgic about it." For the first time she began dating a good deal, at first with men to whom she was introduced by the other girls. She loved her work. "I knew I could be a great pianist. I would often practice eight or ten hours a day, and we'd go to a concert or walk around the city and end up in a restaurant or eating in our rooms. We'd talk all night, and the next day I'd be ready to start all over again."

At the end of the year, plans had been made for all three girls to return and to turn the apartment into a co-operative housing unit. However, her father was adamant (a type of behavior that was markedly unusual for him). He told her she could not return, that life in the city was too "immoral," and that he would not have his daughter living "a life of that kind." He finally convinced her that she would be just as happy at a small progressive college, and she consented to change her plans. After arrival at the school, she felt unhappy and depressed; her interest for her music lessened; and "although I kept practicing, my music was cold, there was nothing of *me* in it anymore." She met a rather emotionally disturbed man whom she quickly married. (On her first view of him through a window, she said to a friend, "That's the man my mother would like me to marry.") In spite of his inability to earn a living, they had three children in rapid succession. She tried desperately to build a strong emotional relationship to him, but like her father, he was afraid of his own warm impulses and the harder she tried, the less he was able to respond. She tried to find close girl friends but could not stand their constant talk of their children and homes, while they soon wearied of her attempts to talk of music, art, and social issues. She did join a chamber music group but found that it was impossible to spend much time with it due to the demands of her family. She found herself becoming more and more easily fatigued and increasingly less interested in anything. Her skill at painting and sculpture also seemed less real and less important to her. Her piano playing became less satisfying. She felt that she could never succeed at anything or get any real enjoyment out of life. Eight years after leaving the group, the first symptoms of Hodgkin's disease were noted.

CHAPTER 16

Repression and Lung Cancer

ALTHOUGH OUR STUDIES THUS FAR have explored a number of emotional patterns and psychological attitudes that seem definitely related to specific types of cancer, the establishment of such a relationship cannot be taken to mean that cancer is a psychosomatic illness. Although the method is completely unknown, there can be little doubt that what actually happens is that a particular emotional state triggers (or is perhaps caused by) specific physical reactions in the body which, in turn, lead to the wild growth of tissue of a particular type in a particular place.

The question was discussed by Dr. A. E. Rakoff of the Jefferson Medical College in Philadelphia at the 1965 Conference of the New York Academy of Sciences we have previously mentioned.

"What meaning can be attributed to these observations?" he asked. And he went on to reply that ". . . the answer may be concerned with mechanisms by which factors can influence biochemical functions. There is now considerable evidence that the endocrine system is at least one important link in integrating the effects of the central nervous system on the biochemical function of various target organs. In our studies demonstrating the influence of psychic factors on ovarian function we have been particularly intrigued by the possibility that such psychically induced hormonal dysfunctions may influence tumorigenesis in certain biologically susceptible individuals, particularly in relationship to those tumors which are believed to be hormonally dependent or hormonally influenced."

Here Dr. Rakoff is entering what is indeed a mysterious field—that of the hundreds of glands the body contains, each of them producing a single hormone or group of hormones, all of them having a fantastically powerful effect on the growth and function of particular tissues, yet most of them constituting an unfathomable puzzle to medical science. The major glands such as the adrenals, the pancreas, the pituitary, have been thoroughly studied and are well understood. But most of the glands of the human anatomy are barely names known to the skilled anatomist, but whose functions are only guessed at and the nature of whose secretions remains unknown. Yet those glands that are well studied are known to alter their functions and change the nature or the quantity of their secretions in response to emotional changes, and the effect of such altered functions is powerful indeed.

Emotional Stress and the Glands

For one obvious example, the secretions of the adrenals directly affect the action of the heart. They respond to emotional stress with minutely increased secretions that strengthen and increase the heartbeat. And it is well known that a perpetual condition of stress which keeps the adrenal glands stimulated can put so much extra strain upon the heart that it can lead to heart attacks.

Dr. Rakoff says that "The growth of certain tissues and organs are known to be relatively dependent on certain trophic hormones. There are observations to suggest that hormonal dependency is applicable not only to normal tissues and organs but also to neoplasms derived from them, such as those of the breasts, prostate and uterus, and of such hormone producing organs as the pituitary, thyroid, adrenal, ovary and testis. This relationship is the basis for the concept of an endocrine influence on the pathogenesis and control of abnormal and neoplastic growth.

"Tumors have been produced experimentally in many tissues which are hormonally responsive by various endocrine manipulations. There have been many clinical observations suggesting that hormonal influences may play a similar role in tumor formation in the human. . . .

"If, indeed, hormonal factors can influence tumorigenesis albeit in ways which are not yet understood, it becomes necessary to examine the thesis that psychic factors may influence hormonal function. This assumption was originally postulated on the basis of numerous clinical observations indicating various types of disturbed hormonal function following psychic traumas. . . . It has been strengthened greatly by the remarkable recent advances in neuroendocrine physiology which indicate that the pituitary and its target endocrine glands are controlled by the hypothalamus, and that the hypothalamic-pituitary mechanism can in turn be influenced by physical or chemical manipulations of various brain structures."

In Dr. Rakoff's view, then, the probable means by which particular emotions might actually give rise to particular types of cancer are these. The emotion (distress, hopelessness, fear, etc.) stimulates a particular gland or group of glands into either greater activity or cessation of activity. In either case, there is dysfunction which affects the particular tissues that are controlled by the glands. The glandular chemical control over the reproduction of these tissues is lost, and the tissues proliferate wildly.

Dr. Rakoff appears to be convinced that the effect of emotions on the glands is responsible for at least some types of cancer of apparently unknown causation. He is not so sure that it applies to other types for which cause is known. Let us, however, take a look at one such type that is perhaps the best known of all and with the best established external cause. We refer, of course, to lung cancer which is known beyond any reasonable doubt to be caused by cigarette smoking. This knowledge does not answer the question, though, of why it is that in any group of heavy cigarette smokers a large proportion will get lung cancer, yet others seem apparently immune.

An interesting study of this disease was made by a Scottish physician and psychologist, David M. Kissen of the University Department of Psychological Medicine, Southern General Hospital, Glasgow, Scotland. Dr. Kissen is not only a psychologist but also a specialist in chest diseases, and so is particularly well qualified for such an investigation.

"My interest in the possibility that psychological factors might play a part in the etiology of lung cancer," he says, "began a number of years ago, when, as a chest physician, I was responsible for a clinic for the diagnosis of chest disorders. One of the first patients who stimulated this interest was a middle-aged married woman who was found to have an inoperable bronchial carcinoma. She had never smoked and during the previous thirty years had lived in a quiet country district free from atmospheric pollution. She presented herself ostensibly as a woman with a healthy physical and emotional background. . . . A more searching interrogation, however, revealed tenuous ties with her aged and ailing parents and emotional conflict about her relationship with them, especially with her father, and with her only sister."

Emotional Conflict

Dr. Kissen's interest in the phenomenon led to a more intensive study, which after a number of years resulted in a particular conclusion:

"The particular feature of personality that I have found to be characteristic among cancer patients I have described as a poor outlet for emotional discharge." He goes on to describe the particular psychological characteristic he means as the "unconscious inability to deal adequately with emotional conflict."

Dr. Kissen studied patients at two surgical chest units and one medical unit, interviewing every patient over the age of 25 before any diagnosis had been made. He was later informed just which chest disorder had been diagnosed and was able to check the diagnoses against his records of interviews.

"By the time I had seen about 150 lung cancer patients and a similar number of non-cancer patients, I began to form a number of hypotheses based on clinical observations. One of these was that lung cancer patients have a significantly diminished outlet for emotional discharge compared with non-cancer patients."

Medical diagnoses were checked against two kinds of psychological findings. In his interviews Dr. Kissen probed whether or not the patient had demonstrated behavior disorders in childhood, reasoning that such disorders, while they might be classified as neuroticism, did give the child a way of discharging anxieties, fears and hostilities that is not possessed by the apparently more normal child. Each patient was also given an objective personality inventory test, with Dr. Kissen looking for the "neuroticism" score, again on the assumption that the patient who demonstrated less "neuroticism" was the one possessing less emotional outlet.

He found a strong statistical correlation between both findings of lack of emotional outlet and subsequent diagnoses of lung cancer.

". . . As a further check, the personality feature was measured in the same way in a second control group of male non-cancer patients from non-chest wards in the same hospitals, approximately age-matched with the cancer patients of the same social classes. The findings were even more striking, significant differences between the lung cancer group and each of the control groups in relation to outlet for emotional discharge being clearly evident."

Dr. Kissen made a further startling finding that might even indicate that psychological factors are more important than the smoking in the development of lung cancer.

"One of the anomalies of lung cancer and smoking statistics is the apparent contradiction in some studies in respect of inhalation of cigarette smoke and lung cancer risk. Indeed some of the figures suggest the possibility *(British Medical Journal,* 1962) that among heavy smokers, non-inhalers may have the greater risk for lung cancer. Comparisons were therefore made between lung cancer inhalers and non-inhalers in respect of outlet for emotional discharge. It was found that non-inhalers had a significantly poorer outlet for emotional discharge than inhalers at all age levels. . . .

"Thus, on the basis of personality, some of the anomalous findings in regard to inhalers and lung cancer may have some rational explanation. Just as, on the basis of personality, a rational explanation is offered for the development of lung cancer in some nonsmokers and light smokers and its nondevelopment in many heavy smokers."

Dr. Kissen does not discard the importance of smoking as a lung cancer cause. He says that "According to information currently available, those most likely to develop lung cancer are heavy cigarette smokers with chronic cough living in urban areas employed in air polluted occupations and a feature of whose personality is a poor outlet for emotional discharge."

He does point out, however, that the psychological characteristics probably play a role in how vulnerable any particular individual is to lung cancer. Pointing out the weakness of warnings about cigarette smoking alone, which are shrugged off by most smokers, Dr. Kissen suggests that the problem is to identify those in the very high risk categories and direct warnings specifically at them. "Preliminary statistical analyses suggest that certain measurable and readily identifiable adverse life situations in childhood and long-standing emotional conflicts in later life may be significant factors predisposing to lung cancer. Such features considered together with the characteristic poor outlet for emotional discharge could conceivably increase considerably the potential contribution of psychological factors to the identification of high risk groups in lung cancer." What it comes down to is that the heavy smoker whose emotions are generally suppressed is particularly vulnerable to this dread disease. The doctor who is aware of this can single out those of his patients who run the greatest risk of contracting lung cancer, and warn them as individuals of their own special vulnerability.

Nothing else seems yet to have had any effect on the plague-like increase in lung cancer. Perhaps such an individual approach might make all the difference.

In any case, Dr. Kissen has opened wide the door to additional, original research into the question of lung cancer and cigarette smoking. Cigarette smoking does cause lung cancer. There is no longer any room for doubt. Yet many cigarette smokers do not contract the disease.

Could the control of the rate of growth of the tissue of the lungs and bronchial tubes be vested in some gland about which we know little or nothing? Is it possible that before the repeated shocks of inhaled tobacco smoke can induce the lung tissue to grow in a wild and uncontrolled manner, it is necessary to knock out the function of one or more glands located elsewhere in the body? And further, is it possible that repression of the emotions and insistence on maintaining a calm demeanor under all circumstances is the psychological attitude that does the glandular damage, thus permitting cigarette smoke to stimulate the worst possible reaction in the lungs?

And where does vitamin A enter into all this? Recently we have seen evidence that vitamin A taken in sufficient quantity can help the lungs to resist the onslaughts of the cancer-causing chemicals in tobacco smoke. Does it do this directly or does it do it by maintaining the health of some gland that otherwise might be put out of commission by destructive emotional attitudes?

We cannot say that any of these things are so. What we do say is that the studies already made of the relation between emotions and cancer make it imperative that the above questions and many others be investigated by competent scientists and ultimately answered.

CHAPTER 17

Personal Loss and the Lymphatics

IN 1952 A MEDICAL PSYCHIATRIST at the University of Rochester School of Medicine wrote a paper based on his professional experience that was so startling at that time that the journal *Psychosomatic Medicine* held it for two years before finally publishing it in 1954. The doctor was William A. Greene, Jr. and his paper was titled "Psychological Factors and Reticuloendothelial Disease." Behind the conservative technical title there lay a radical study of the personalities and personal histories of a group of men who had contracted either lymphomas or leukemias, which is to say cancer of the lymphatics whether it was manifested as tumors of the lymph glands themselves, or derangement of their blood-forming function causing wild overproduction of the white blood cells.

In an introduction to his paper, Dr. Greene attributes the idea for his study to earlier work by Dr. Hans Selye which suggested that non-specific stress such as psychological stress could be the source of disease. Selye had already suggested that the lymphatics were among the organs that could be affected by such stress, and so Dr. Greene undertook to make a study of consecutive patients admitted to hospitals in Rochester, New York, with various forms of cancer of the lymphatics. This first study published by Dr. Greene dealt with 20 males ranging in age from 3 years to 78. The group included 3 boys below the age of 5 and 1 adolescent.

"In all 20 cases," says Dr. Greene, "the development and recognition of the lymphoma or leukemia occurred while the patient was having to adjust to a loss of (psychological) support. This included loss of significant object relationships. In 17 patients, this loss involved varying degrees of separation from a parent-figure, usually mother or a mother-figure. This was most frequently due to death of the parent, but was manifest in other cases by desertion or by birth of a sibling rival . . ." (A sibling rival is a younger brother or sister whose arrival on the scene is interpreted as causing the loss of parental love and attention.)

Object Loss

Although he had looked for a particular type of personality that might lead to an increased possibility of contracting cancer of the lymph gland system, Dr. Greene could not find one. He states that there was no common personality type, nor was there even a characteristic conflict situation for these patients as a group. Regardless of their differing personalities, however, these patients all showed symptoms of anxiety reaction and depression which had usually been present for months before any organic disease had manifested itself. It was also common to find loss of appetite, vomiting and pain in the gastro-intestinal system for months or years in the past history but without any known organic cause.

Numerous case histories that demonstrate both the variety of personality types and the similarity of circumstance in the personal history that is described as "object loss" are cited. Let us examine a few of them:

A three and a half-year-old boy described by his parents as being unusually "clinging" was apparently in normal health and not unusual except for his undue attachment to his parents and his home and personal belongings. "Four months ago the house in which the family was living burned down. It had caught on fire from the house next door which also burned down the same night. No one was burned or injured, but all the family's possessions, including the patient's toys, bed and clothes were destroyed. . . . Following the fire, the family moved in with the paternal grandparents, where the parents and patient occupied one room as they had done at home. Since making this move, the patient had been wetting the bed again each night. (This is a well-known sign of emotional anxiety.) A month after the fire, the older 18-year-old son left home to join the army."

Four months after the fire, the child was admitted to the hospital as a leukemia patient. Dr. Greene points out that while he had obviously had a strong emotional reaction to losing his home, his toys and later his older brother, his emotion had not been overtly expressed and could only be guessed at from the fact that he was wetting his bed. The child next door who was constantly screaming and crying as a result of his fright and deprivation (his house had also burned down) developed no illness.

Dr. Greene's case five was a man whose entire family had died when he was relatively young, except for his only daughter, who also died when he was 47 years old. Several months after the death of his daughter, when he had been left alone in the world, he consulted a doctor for back pain and was recognized to have leukemia.

Case eight was that of a 15-year-old boy who apparently had a bad relationship with his family but clung to the parochial school to which he was sent. At the age of 14, on graduation from the grade school level, he was shifted to a trade school, and in the same year his closest friend died suddenly of rheumatic heart disease. The boy developed sarcoma of the lymphatics.

Case nine was that of a 48-year-old man who apparently was not inordinately attached to his wife and two children, but had a deep emotional dependence on his mother. When his mother died he began to get a sour stomach and heartburn and in two years' time he was found to have contracted leukemia.

Dr. Greene's case twelve is especially interesting to us. In this case, the patient who was involved was apparently dependent on support in the strict economic sense. He had always lived with his mother who had taken care of him. "She had died three years before the patient came to the hospital. He then lived with his older sister. Her husband had had a heart attack the year before, necessitating his stopping work and staying at home." The burden of supporting the family fell on the patient, with no one left in the world who could or would take care of him. "The patient was admitted with complaints of weakness, fatigue, and pain in the inguinal region for four months. Physical examination showed no abnormality, but study of his blood and bone marrow showed myelocytic leukemia."

"A 37-year-old man had always had a close relationship with his mother and distant relationship with his father. After the war he returned to his home, his first experience there since his mother's death, which occurred while he was in the service. He invested all his savings in a theatrical venture which failed. At the same time he found out that his girl friend was already married. He became increasingly depressed, weeping without apparent provocation, and talking of how worthless and unsuccessful he was. After a year of these symptoms an enlarging cervical node was first recognized, and this, on biopsy, showed Hodgkin's disease."

In discussing these cases, Dr. Greene attempts to consider whether the psychological stresses involved can be the cause of the development of the illness. He is inclined to doubt that the stress alone could be a complete cause. "We do not think that the current psychological stresses ought to be considered as the causes of the lymphoma or the leukemia, but only as one factor, perhaps the precipitating factor contributing to a disease with this type of pathology in these individuals."

In other words, to put the question in our more general terms, he does not believe that unhappiness in itself is enough to cause cancer, but he has found evidence that the unhappiness is one of the important factors involved in the development of cancer. This implies, of course, that in a happier personality the other physical causes would have less chance of undermining the health and ultimately killing the person.

We consider point number two of Dr. Greene's summary the most important: "In all of these cases, the symptoms and the recognition of the disease occurred while the patient was having to adjust to multiple stresses, which arose from multiple sources. In 17 of the 20 patients, these stresses included separation from a significant person, father, mother, wife, or other mother-figure, usually by death. Such separation also occurred with advent of sibling rivals as actual siblings or offspring. Frequently there were coincidental problems in life adjustment related to work, infection, injury, or operation."

At the time he wrote this first study in 1952, Dr. Greene was by no means certain whether he had actually found something important or was just kidding himself. By 1955, however, when he published a second study regarding the occurrence of the same forms of cancer in women, he was much more certain that he was right. In the first study he was careful to point out that the entire relationship might be nothing more than coincidence. By the time the second study had been completed, he had enough case histories compiled and had found such startling similarities in the psychological stress involved, that there was no longer any room for doubt.

CHAPTER 18

Mothers, Daughters and Leukemia

IT WAS POINTED OUT in the last chapter that when Dr. William A. Greene, Jr. published his first paper regarding a relationship between malignant disease of the lymphatics and the loss of support in the psychological sense, he was by no means sure of the validity of his conclusion. His study had involved only 20 males, 3 boys and 17 men. It had turned out to be highly suggestive, but could hardly be called conclusive.

Dr. Greene was careful to point out that in a sample as limited as the one he had been able to deal with, the psychological similarities might be nothing more than coincidence.

By 1955, Dr. Greene and two collaborators, Lawrence Young, M.D. and Scott Swisher, M.D., had made a second study of 32 women under the same circumstances.

There was no longer any possibility of coincidence. Dr. Greene could feel with much greater confidence that that he had really hit upon something.

The second female study was described in *Psychosomatic Medicine* (XVIII, 4, 1956).

All 32 women were either under care of the hematology section of the University of Rochester School of Medicine or had at least been examined by that section. The diagnoses of their conditions in every case were clinical, made or confirmed by appropriate examinations of blood, bone marrow, or biopsy material. 19 had leukemia and 13 lymphoma.

Although it proved impossible to find a single definable type of personality among all 32 patients, the researchers were able to isolate four distinctive personality characteristics. The patients were then divided into 4 groups according to their personality traits. The first group included 12 women classified as "mother" personalities. These women not only cared for their own children, but cared for foster children, other adults, and the sick. The second group, consisting of 5 women, were characterized as "manly." They were employed in masculine type jobs and were relatively self-sufficient. The remaining 15 patients were basically dependent and clinging personalities, but were divided into 2 groups because 9 of the women displayed a false independent and isolationist tendency.

All of these patients, it is stated by Dr. Greene and his associates, emphasized that in the past they had been self-sufficient and independent of help from others, particularly doctors. Another characteristic they shared was a general inability to express anger. It had been their habit to relieve emotional tensions through hard physical work or some kind of gross activity, at which they had generally been capable and effective.

"While the patients of these four groups present quite diversified personality characteristics, we have the impression that underlying all of these manifestations may have been a basic unresolved attachment to the mother." Most of the women had been physically healthy in the past. Their main symptoms of disease had been episodes of upper gastrointestinal distress such as nausea, vomiting and loss of appetite. None of them ever had a peptic ulcer.

Traumatic Separations

Because, in the male study reported in the last chapter, it is found that the stress of separation was a possible psychological stimulus to cancer of the lymphatics, the women of the second report were also questioned intensively to determine what kinds of emotional stress they had been subjected to in the period up to four years before the apparent onset of their disease.

It was found that "these stresses have included loss by death, or the threat of death incident to a major illness, of a significant person—mother, father, husband or child." The threat of separation from active life as represented symbolically by the menopause was another important stress.

Of the above types of losses, real or threatened, it was found that one or more had occurred to 30 of the 32 patients being studied during the four-year period before the onset of their malignant disease. In 16 patients there were three or more such episodes, in 9 patients there were two.

The remaining 2 patients did not experience an emotional loss or separation of the type we have described, but suffered severe emotional strain in the year before they became ill.

Patients Believe Sadness Caused Disease

"A striking finding has been the fact that in this series of 32 women patients with leukemia or lymphoma, 19 consciously related the distressing effect to a preceding loss or separation with accompanying sadness or 'nervousness.' Five related the effect to activity or fatigue in relation to an obvious separation . . . only eight of the women attributed their distressing effect to the current illness."

So we see that the women themselves, in a ratio of three to one, were convinced that their emotional distress caused the disease rather than the reverse.

One difference between the women who had contracted lymphomas and people studied in relation to other forms of cancer was that there was a singular absence of feelings of guilt among the women with leukemia or lymphoma. Instead of guilt, there was an apparent dominating feeling of shame which was harbored by the patients long before they became physically ill. The authors believe there is a definite significance in the psychological difference and that there is a distinct possibility that shame will lead to lymphoma or leukemia whereas guilt will end in other types of neoplasms.

Highly significant to us, this is the first paper on the subject we have seen that raises the possibility that psychological treatment can actually be effective in the management of cancer. Successful treatment of a cancer patient not only involves the medical procedure the doctor employs, but also patient relationships with his doctor and within his family. It is an indication that if the life of the patient can be re-arranged in such a way that separation is either compensated for or no longer threatened, the patient will have a far better response to the physical therapy employed and will not have as great a tendency to relapse.

Thus another group of investigators have added their evidence to the growing store of information about the relationship between emotions and cancer. I'm beginning to suspect that some day, when it is all correlated and tallied up by some mathematician, it will be found that in many thousands of cases of cancer, practically all were uniformly preceded by psychological blows, usually psychic losses, and a state of profound sadness or depression.

CHAPTER 19

Nuns Live Longer

"THE SISTERS OF AMERICA are the healthiest, most dedicated, best-educated, longest-living group of women in America today." So said J. T. Nix, M.D., Ph.D., a physician and surgeon who has devoted many years to studying the health problems of nuns as well as treating them. The details and conclusions of his study give us a fortunate opportunity to begin examining the positive side of the relationship between emotional states and cancer.

Nuns do not lead lives of perfect emotional health, of course, any more than they lead lives of perfect physical health. All the same, "nuns have their breast cancers 15 years later than other American white single women." This statement was made by Dr. Nix in a speech to the National Conference of Major Religious Superiors in August, 1966. It was based on an analysis he had made of the causes of death of over 3,000 nuns out of a total nun population of 108,000 during the years 1963, 1964 and 1965. The study was so thorough as to place the fact beyond argument. Nuns are healthier than other women and nuns live longer than other women. The average age of death was found to be 76. Among those who died of cancer, by far the leading cause was cancer of the breast which might perhaps be expected among women who have renounced the function of motherhood and have led celibate lives. Yet even so, such cancers occur far, far later in life than they do to equivalent unmarried and married women of the general population.

It will be recalled that in earlier chapters we have found time and again that there is a relationship between the development of cancer and the loss of a sense of purpose in living. Whether it be forced retirement from a career or the loss of a person to whom a woman's life has been devoted, whether the personality be a saintly one or self-centered and selfish, we have found time after time that dedication and devotion seem to have kept particular people well, while they lapsed into illness upon loss of that to which they were dedicated.

Does this mean that every person must find a way to dedicate his life or else he will become sick? Not at all. Most people have no such demand within their personalities. Most people are able to concern their lives with relatively small affairs, looking for pleasure and accepting sadness or pain, but living always within the framework of their own needs and desires. There are only a relatively small number of people who seem unable to experience life directly, but feel great joys and sorrows only in terms of what is happening to some other loved person rather than themselves. Or, of course, it might be an artistic career or a business that gains all the attention and devotion. People who must devote themselves to something outside their own beings are comparatively rare birds. And we have seen that it is from this less usual kind of person that many candidates for cancer are recruited.

It would also seem to be apparent that women who enter the religious life—particularly Catholics who take the veil, thus giving up many of the most important pleasures and fulfillments of normal living—would also be of this particular type with a particularly strong need to live lives of devotion to something outside themselves.

If we put together these two facts, a hasty judgment might suppose that nuns could be expected to have a higher than average rate of cancer. Yet we have the word of Dr. Nix for it that the exact reverse is true. Nuns are surely drawn from the cancer-prone of personalities, yet they live longer rather than shorter lives, develop less rather than more cancer, and when they do develop cancer, do so at a substantially older age.

Psychologically, we believe, there are two important reasons for this. First, the nun has ready-made for her not only an opportunity but an obligation to devote her life to service. And we have already seen that such intense devotion has gone a long way to maintain health in people who might well be analyzed as cancer-prone.

Secondly, the nun's area of devotion is far bigger than a single person, a business or a career. Where other women of the same devotional type find in middle age that their families have grown up and left them, or their parents or husband have died, and they seem to have nothing left to make demands upon them, for the nun, the church, the religion, and people in general go on forever. Therefore she has no reason for a sudden loss of interest in living and a sudden loss of resistance to disease occurring in her fifties or sixties.

Consider this statement by Dr. Nix from a medical care manual titled "Health to Match Her Dedication":

"Each sister must have a goal in life and a method of achieving it. Her ideal personality reflects a proper balance of work, prayer, love of her religious family, and recreation. She needs time to think, time to dream, and time to achieve. She also has the need to be needed, a sense of belonging, that dignity of personal accomplishment which is gained through a feeling of security at home and at work. . . .

"Each sister enters the novitiate with a different personality reflecting her home environment. Her personality is fundamentally altered by a new set of values required in the novitiate. In religious life the community superior assumes the psychological role of parent. Psychological necessities are not luxuries. She needs solitude, the solicitude of her superiors, a sense of personal integrity, an awareness of her own ability, and a sense of self-determination to give her a contented heart.

"Each sister's health mirrors her environment; the diseases of stress are nature's revenge for the morbidity of tension. . . .

"Time can be bought by dedication to efficiency and delegation to the laity. An active apostolate, radiating spiritual and professional superiority, needs not only physical stamina but also vocational assignment through scientific methods. Our primary interest must always be the effect of the job on the sister, not the effect of the sister on the job."

The above statement by Dr. Nix reflects a growing awareness by the Catholic church that the nun must find fulfillment in her work. While it is hard to pin down the exact degree of happiness such fulfillment represents, it certainly can be said to reduce unhappiness or perhaps make unhappiness impossible.

It should be mentioned at this point that nuns also tend, in the present day, to eat a better diet than women of the general population. Menus are planned by trained dieticians who see to it that they contain a good supply of vitamins and minerals, substantial proportions of raw foods, and that they minimize or entirely avoid rich desserts and sugary foods. Such diets, avoiding the refined carbohydrates that destroy the vitamin B in one's system, also supply more of the B complex vitamins, through which they have a highly beneficial effect on the nerves and emotions. The vitamin B status of the blood is very often the only difference between an energetic and happy person and one who is disturbed and anxious. It is both through careful occupational assignment, therefore, and a healthful way of living, that nuns are encouraged to greater fulfillment and emotional health.

We can thus see why it should be so that even though nuns are single women who never experience motherhood and therefore lie in the particular group that is especially prone to contract cancer of the breast, they only do so at a far later age—a full 15 years later than single women of the general population. Yet if their lives are so wholesome and their emotional health so good, why do they ever contract it?

One answer, we believe, lies in the fact that even though they have no formal retirement, in effect nuns also lose the objects on which their devotion is centered, though at a later age. Writing about nuns over the age of 65, Dr. Nix says that: "We anticipate that five per cent of the sisters between ages 65 and 74 years will be partially inactive, and that 20 per cent of the sisters 75 years of age or older will be inactive and immobile. In all probability, sisters 65 years and older will have three times the number of days of disabling illness with restricted activity per person per year than the sisters in the 15 to 40 year age group."

As a practical administrative matter, this means that as nuns get older—past 65 specifically—their duties are reduced. They are expected to let others take care of them and are deprived of the obligation and privilege of taking care of others. According to a study made by Sister Mary Carol Tate, "Seventy-five per cent of the communities cared for elderly sisters at the Mother House while one community utilized a convent-rest home."

Even though it comes later in life and is more gradual, retirement and loss of an object for her devotion eventually strikes the elderly nun just as it does other people. When that stage is reached, we may suppose, she then becomes more likely to contract cancer of the breast, just like her lay sister who has lost her husband or an only child.

CHAPTER 20

The Exaltation of Walking

EARLIER CHAPTERS HAVE PRESENTED what I consider a convincing case for a connection between cancer and hopelessness, despair and allied emotional patterns indicative of extreme unhappiness. And on the contrary, I have shown in the case of nuns that a way of life that can stave off unhappiness and never allow it to reach an extreme leads to an incidence of cancer that is far lower than the population average.

Not all of us can be nuns, however. Instead of having techniques ready made for us, we have to find our own ways that will enable us to lift our spirits no matter how discouraging circumstances may be.

One way that has always worked for me has been walking.

In the *Medical Record*, August 17, 1938, Norman D. Mattison, M.D. speaks of health, as follows: "If a person is not ill, has no symptoms to be diagnosed as characteristic of disease, can go about ordinary affairs with reasonable efficiency, he is considered 'well.' That an individual should experience the sensation of positive well-being, of happy competence for life, the joy of performance, is so rare that we have no definite terms to express these sensations or the state of physical health that assures them. Any description of perfect and positive health, therefore, is literary in character."

Actually, there is a term that can be applied to such a state: "euphoria." It means a terrifically wonderful feeling of well-being, when one is purring, when the soul is singing, when one can feel it in every part of the body, right into his fingertips. The French use the word *euphoria* a good deal, but it is so new as far as English is concerned that you will not find it in the ordinary English dictionary. The syllable *eu* of this word is from the Greek and means "well." It is found in such a word as "eudaemonism," a system of ethics that regards happiness as the chief end to be attained; "eugenic," which literally means "well-born"; "eulogy," praise; "euphemism," a pleasing expression; "euphonic," pleasantness of sounds; and of course the word "beautiful," where the *eu* is hidden in the middle.

I might also say that thinking along these lines, we must not define health as a mere absence of disease. There must be something more.

Ah, euphoria! I had it once when I was eight years old. I can see myself even now, standing in front of a tenement in New York City. It was the first warm day of spring—early in May. The air was balmy and it was the first time I was able to go out without a coat. I can still remember my very white shirt standing out in the drab surroundings. There was a deep-souled, overcharged feeling of well-being that came after months of pent-up inactivity. I can still see myself standing there—a short thin lad, but full of glowing euphoria. It is a recollection that will stay with me always.

Another time I can remember having euphoria was at the age of about 15. In the late afternoon I was returning from high school and stood on the 59th Street platform waiting for the Ninth Avenue elevated train. I was up in the air and I must have had a good day at school. I felt as if I were the happiest boy in the world. My soul was singing within me.

But a few years ago I had a full three weeks of euphoria. It was during a five-week tour of Europe. The trip began in London, went to Amsterdam, Stockholm, Copenhagen, Hamburg, Hanover, Stuttgart, Zurich, Vienna, Milan and Paris. Every day for five solid weeks, I walked five hours—rain or shine. When seeing a foreign city I love to walk in its streets, look in store windows and observe the people, the architecture, the sculptured street art, and so forth.

The euphoria came after the second week. In Hanover, I felt it in the late afternoon after about three hours of walking—a wonderful feeling of exhilaration when the physical side of the body touches and merges with the spiritual, when I felt like singing and dancing. Now I can see why the savages dance and shout. They become so overcharged with oxygen from being outdoors and moving about that it gives them a strongly euphoric feeling, and then they have to express their happiness by jumping about. Our square dancing is pink tea in comparison.

In Hanover, Germany I met H. A. Schweigert, M.D., who has done research in cancer. When I told him of my experience he commented that since the time of his research showing that in all cancerous tissue there is a deficiency of oxygen, he has been walking for one hour every morning.

This was corroborated about a year later when I read that at a Chicago meeting of the Radiological Society of North America, (*Science News Letter*, Dec. 7, 1963) a promising treatment of cancer with oxygen was described in patients with incurable tumors. Although there were few cures, there was a dramatic reduction of pain in most cases. The treatment forces oxygen into cells that lack a normal supply of it.

My own determined desire to walk every day became like a drug! My body craved it! I will never forget the day in Stuttgart when it was raining cats and dogs, but I was not deterred. I took a taxi to the imposing two-block-long *Bahnhof*, or railroad station, and there I walked and walked, until the weather cleared up. And I enjoyed walking there, looking into all the shop windows in the station, observing the general hustle and bustle of people coming and going, and being a part of the traveling atmosphere.

Ah, euphoria! Here I was, about 65 years old and feeling like that day in May when I was only 8. In fact, I think I felt better. I was taking my vitamin E every day, the vitamin that oxygenates the tissues, and the exercise pushed the effect of the vitamin E until it penetrated into the deepest crevices of my body.

This feeling stayed with me until I came home where I went back to my one-hour-a-day walking routine, due to the work I have to get done. And I haven't had a single day of euphoria since I've been back, although in Atlantic City a few weeks ago I walked for 6½ hours one day, two hours of which I walked barefoot along the beach. I tried to recapture euphoria a month ago by taking a 4½-hour hike from our farm to Limeport, over the mountain, but I find in my own case that euphoria comes only after weeks of daily doses of heavy oxygenation.

But please don't misunderstand me. Euphoria is one thing and just feeling good is another. I feel great, but it isn't euphoria.

There was the case of an old man in New York City, a Syrian who reached the age of 116. When asked to what he attributed it, he said that for the last 30 years or so he had been on the go all day long. He kept walking and moving about because he sensed something wonderful about it—evidently a feeling of euphoria.

When I get to be about 80, I will do the same, but with two or three secretaries to keep me company and to take notes.

Euphoria is another way of saying, the nth degree of happiness.

Hill Walking

I have recently had an experience in connection with my daily walking program that is worth relating. As my readers know, for the last 4 or 5 years I have been walking, an hour a day, with wonderful benefit to my physical condition, especially with a reduction of my pulse from about 85 to about 65 to 72. But something occurred last winter which indicated to me that there is more to walking than just walking.

We had taken a house for the entire winter in Palm Beach so that I would be able to do my walking every day. But it did not work out the way I expected. I did my regular stint of walking every day but somehow I did not feel that I was thriving on it as well as I did at home. For one thing, my speaking voice became weaker. I didn't have my blood pressure taken while there, but when we came home and I had it checked I found that it had jumped from 120 to about 140.

Well, this called for some thinking, but for the time being nothing came of it. About a month later I had my blood pressure taken again, but this time it had gone back to normal, namely 120. And my voice had come back to its normal pitch. You can believe that I immediately set myself to do some tall thinking. It did not take me long to get what I believed to be the answer for what had happened in Florida.

Palm Beach is as flat as a pancake, whereas at home I walked among gently rolling hills. The effort of pushing upward while walking evidently has much more beneficial effect than walking on the flat. Besides, at home I slept on the second floor, and went up and down stairs many times a day. In Palm Beach our rented house was a one-story affair.

So I realized at once that walking up hill is far more healthful than walking on a flat surface. It so happens that there are some steep hills near our farm, which up to now I had been avoiding. Now I began to lay out a daily walk of one hour that took in only the steepest hills I could find. The effect? Amazing! And me a heart case that was turned down for life insurance in 1953 (Metropolitan Life Insurance Co.). I am writing this 15 years later.

I took these hills with a confidence engendered by taking large protective doses of vitamin E (1,200 milligrams daily of mixed tocopherols).

Alfred Bendiner, a well-known Philadelphia architect, in his "Sketchbook" has described the Manayunk area of Philadelphia. Living there means arduous hill-climbing. Here is what Bendiner says about it, in the *Sunday Bulletin Magazine* (March 11, 1962).

"People used to get enough exercise just walking those hard hills. If you know your way around, there are 'the Blocks' and 'Little Germany' and the closely knit groups of Italians and other minorities who have lived to be over 80 and who remember the good old days when you had to walk up and down, instead of crowding the curbs with Cadillacs."

While in Germany recently, a friend told me about a doctor who was suffering from high blood pressure. He cured himself by walking to the top of mountains with the aid of two long sticks. Now he says, "I have

4 feet." He has so conditioned himself that he can outclimb far younger persons.

If you are deciding on a vacation spot pick out a hilly region. If you wish to move to a new location, choose a hilly one. Your children will grow up healthier there.

I was recently reading *The Citadel* by A. J. Cronin, and came to an interesting passage. A woman is berating a doctor who seldom prescribed medicines. She says, "Go on with you, Doctor. He's reg'lar quee-ar. Mostly he don't give medicine at all. Why when Megan Rhys Morgan, what's had to have medicine all her life, went to him, he told her to walk two miles up the mountain every day and stop boggin' herself with hogwash" (meaning medicine). More physicians should suggest hill walking to their patients and they will dispense less medicine.

We are told that in Bulgaria and Yugoslavia there are sections where people live to be very old. Usually the reason is given that these people drink a certain kind of sour milk that teems with beneficial microscopic organisms. I wonder if these people live in mountainous regions and have hardened their bodies by walking daily in steep hills. Perhaps it is the effect of both. However, it would be a good thing if some research organization compared the death rates and the extent of chronic disease as between hilly and flat regions.

When I began to walk my hills I took it easy at first because of my heart condition. I would stop to rest for 20 or 30 seconds whenever I felt too tired to go on with comfort. At the beginning I would have to stop 10 times before reaching the top of a hill. On the first day I had to go to bed for 3 hours after I returned from the walk—I was so fatigued. Within two days I did not require any nap at all. In fact, on one of these days I experienced a wonderful feeling of euphoria which I had not felt in a long time . . . a strange, pleasant exhilaration.

Gradually I was able to go higher on a hill before making my first stop. I figured that by the end of the summer I would be able to make all the hills without any stops at all. But I was able to accomplish this by June 28, approximately a month and a half after I began my hill-walking regimen.

The first time that I made the longest hill without stopping, I must have been helped along by some church singing that came out of the Salisbury Church that is located at the top. It seemed to be inspired with a divine fire. They were singing "O Living Bread from Heaven." I stood transfixed, drinking it in with tremendous enjoyment. If you wish to experience a heavenly feeling, walk up a long hill and suddenly come upon a church at the top with singing voices coming forth. Moses walked up to Mt. Sinai to get the Ten Commandments. Christ walked up to the mount to give His famous sermon. Walking hills will lift you up in more senses than one.

One particular week-day I walked up this hill and the church of course was empty, but the door being invitingly open, I went in. What a wonderful feeling surged over me. Oh, how I wished a minister was there that I could communicate my feelings to him. Churches should be on top of hills and the people should walk up to worship.

Walking, whether on the flat or in hills, is of great benefit to one's spirits. It drives away fears. It contributes towards a happy feeling. At least I find it so.

As far as the effect of exercise on cancer is concerned, there appeared a report in *The Dog World* for June, 1960, part of which I will quote: "Animals allowed to exercise freely are more resistant to the growth of cancer than those kept inactive in small individual cages." This was reported to the Federation of American Societies for Experimental Biology by a trio of researchers from the Jefferson Medical College, Philadelphia. The inhibition (reduction) of cancer growth was even more marked in animals forced to do strenuous exercise such as running for many miles each day or swimming for hours in a tank.

The animals used in the tests were rats with transplanted cancers. The rats forced to lead completely indolent lives carried cancer 5 to 10 times the weight of those in the over-exercised animals, and in some cases the cancers in the exercised rats appeared to have disappeared completely.

In closing this chapter I would like to suggest that cancer hospitals should be pleasant places set on top of mountains where one could see for miles around, where the air is rarefied and exhilarating and where the patients will have the spiritual pleasure of being on top of a mountain.

There should also be vegetable gardens tended by the patients.

CHAPTER 21

A Healthy Mind in a Healthy Body

IF YOU HAVE EVER WORN a pair of shoes that were too tight, then you are all too familiar with the phenomenon that pain or discomfort in your feet can cause you to quarrel with your friends, become hypercritical of your children, be impatient, antagonistic, or so sensitive that you can burst into tears on little or no provocation. It is a clear and understandable demonstration of the indisputable fact that ill health or dysfunction anywhere in your body is going to have some effect on how you think and how you behave. To some degree, it is going to warp your emotions and your mentality away from the normal, the normal being the cheerful, optimistic and clear-thinking mentality that is characteristic of those in perfect health.

So in giving consideration to ways to avoid the depressed and jaundiced state of mind that we have seen can predispose to various types of cancer, it would be sinful to neglect the question of general health. While overall health is not the only element involved in emotional patterns by any means, it nevertheless does and must play an important role. And if you wish to guard your own mentality against dangerous yet subtle distortions of which you might not be aware yourself, one of your best shields will be found to be the health of your own body. Nor is that a question that is up to your doctor. His role—at least as he sees it—is to cure or alleviate sickness. Building better health is very much your own problem.

To help people find the kind of superb health that enables them to resist all kinds of disease, I have developed a general program that has been previously published as the PREVENTION Program. There is hardly a person alive who could not benefit his health in some way by following every item of this program. Space does not permit its full reproduction here, but here are a number of the highlights of special interest to those concerned with the interrelationship between physical and mental health.

Alcohol. Recent researchers have proven that it is a fallacy to believe that a small amount of alcohol every day is good for older persons, that it opens up the arteries. It opens them up only temporarily but its after-effect is harmful. Alcohol uses up vitamin B in the body and is harmful to the nervous system. While some people seem to get along on a small amount of liquor every day, they would get along much better without it.

Bread. Bread is not the staff of life and in the PREVENTION system there is no place for it, even though it be made of wholewheat. It is fattening, constipating, ferments in the stomach, causes heart symptoms in many heart patients, celiac disease in children, rickets if there is not sufficient vitamin D, is a factor in causing colds, stuffed noses, and many other conditions too numerous to mention here. Try a breadless and grainless diet for a month and see what it will do for you. This also means cutting out cakes, spaghetti, noodles, gravy, etc. By cutting out this form of starch you will have to fill up on more vegetables.

Coffee and Tea. Both are very harmful, but usually do not show their effects until in later years. The tottering gait of a senile old person is due greatly to drinking coffee or tea. The caffeine in coffee and the phylline of tea destroy nerve cells, and in later years play havoc with the memory. They also lower the blood sugar. There is rose hip tea, peppermint, and many herb teas that make excellent drinks, including —Postum.

Eggs. Eggs are the number one protein, and should even be consumed by heart cases, as the egg contains lecithin which is the antidote to cholesterol. It has been found that poor children who can't afford eggs get rheumatoid arthritis where wealthier children do not.

Meat. We are in favor of a diet containing plenty of meats but not of the smoked or processed kinds—no delicatessen. We do not favor vegetarianism.

Milk. We are not in favor of adults drinking milk. There are many conditions and allergies that come from milk drinking. It is too complicated a subject to cover here, but my advice to adults is . . . no milk, butter, cheese, ice cream, etc. A trial will convince you.

Organically Raised Food. As far as possible, make an attempt to raise your own food organically, which means without chemical fertilizers or poison sprays. In the organic method compost fertilizers are used, made of manure, grass clippings, weeds and other plant and animal residues. A small garden will be enough to raise all the vegetables for the average family.

Foods raised with chemical fertilizers have less vitamins and minerals, as well as dangerous amounts of poisonous insecticide residues which are harmful to the health. But if you have to eat commercially produced food, our system of taking vitamins and food supplements will protect you.

Protein. PREVENTION favors a diet high in protein and low in carbohydrates. The latest medical researches show that a diet high in carbohydrates can lead to a heart attack. The organs of our body are practically entirely composed of protein, and meat and fish are the best source of it.

Salt. It is common medical practice to limit salt consumption in heart cases, kidney disease, dropsy, blood pressure, etc. There is also evidence that it can cause deafness, sinus trouble, obesity, hives, etc. Ample salt is contained in food without adding any more.

Seeds. PREVENTION advocates the eating of a certain amount of seeds raw and unsalted. This includes sunflower seeds, corn, nuts, pears, etc. The seed is alive and contains powerful nutritional living substances such as vitamins, enzymes, etc. Remember if such a seed is planted it will grow.

Sleep. One should sleep on a hard mattress, or place a board under a soft one. If one has pains in the neck, try sleeping without a pillow.

Sugar. Sugar, besides being fattening, has been found to be dangerous for heart cases as it distorts the calcium-phosphorus relationship in the blood, and strange as it may seem, if consumed in large amounts, it creates low blood sugar which could lead to mental and other troubles. There should be no candy, cake, pie, ice cream, soft drinks, chewing gum, etc. in the diet. The best form is the natural sugar found in fruits and some vegetables. Honey in moderation. We do not favor brown sugar either, nor do we recommend saccharin, sucaryl, or any of the other synthetic chemical sweeteners.

Tobacco. We are against the use of tobacco in any form. It uses up vitamin C in the body. Not only is it a factor in causing cancer of the lungs, but it is bad for the heart, the functioning of the brain, the eyes, nervous system, blood pressure, pulse, lower extremities, etc. Tobacco leaves have been sprayed with many poisonous chemicals, thus adding to the toxic effect of the nicotine.

Unsaturated Fatty Acids. These are esssential from a nutrition standpoint, because the body cannot manufacture them. They occur in unprocessed natural fats chiefly of vegetable origin, such as cereal and vegetable oils like salad oils, olive oil, corn oil, peanut oil. Also in avocadoes, nuts and, of course, sunflower seeds and other seeds. These are the fatty substances which are powerful to prevent cholesterol deposits in the blood vessels.

We advise keeping to a minimum the animal fat in the diet, and shunning hydrogenated fats (solid ones like margarine and the canned shortenings) . Salad oils and other sources of vegetable fats are good for you.

Vitamin and Mineral Supplements. Even if you eat the best possible diet, you do not obtain enough vitamins and minerals for robust health from today's refined and chemically fertilized foods. Much of the fresh food you eat has lost most of its vitamin content during the long shipping process before it reaches your grocery. We advise you to supplement your diet with vitamins and minerals from natural sources. Take them with your meals. They are food.

Vitamin A and D—most plentiful in fish liver oil. Make certain the product you buy is natural, not synthetic.

Vitamin B—Take brewer's yeast and/or desiccated liver for all the vitamins of the B complex. Wheat germ is also very rich in vitamin B, as are sunflower seeds. It is much better for you to get your B vitamins from a natural source like this than to take just one or several in a synthetic vitamin preparation.

Vitamin C—Rose hips contain more vitamin C per gram than any other food. You must have vitamin C every day. Your body cannot store it. Take a rose hip preparation for vitamin C.

Vitamin E—This occurs in whole grain foods, chiefly. If you have been eating refined cereals you are undoubtedly deficient in vitamin E. We believe that everyone should take vitamin E as a daily food supplement. Use the supplement from a natural vegetable source, not the synthetic.

Vitamin E is a most important vitamin which has been almost entirely removed from our foods by processing.

Bone Meal. Lack of calcium, phosphorus and other minerals is one of our most serious diet deficiencies, resulting in tooth decay and scores of other ailments. Bone meal provides them in completely natural form. Take bone meal every day—either in tablets or powdered.

Bone meal prevents tooth cavities, it strengthens the bones against fracture and it has a beneficial effect on the pulse.

Walking and Exercise. A most important function of your body which cannot be neglected if you would be healthy is exercise. For those who work at sedentary occupations especially, it is essential you exercise in the open air every day. Walking is especially good for you, bringing all the muscles into play and providing oxygen for the tissues at a rapid rate. One should walk at least an hour a day, unless one can do some regular exercise equivalent to it each day, not only at weekends.

Walking regulates the glands, reduces a high pulse and is extremely valuable in heart conditions. The average heart case should gradually get used to walking at least an hour a day.

Hill walking is at least 5 times more beneficial than walking on the flat, and climbing stairs is terrific for body health. A prominent physician recently advised walking before breakfast.

Water-Softeners. If you use a water-softener, have it work on the hot water faucet only. To drink artificially softened water is extremely dangerous. The water softening process produces a chemical action in which calcium and magnesium are removed and sodium is placed into the water. This is the equivalent of adding salt to the water. Calcium and magnesium are both of tremendous value to good health.

Following the above rules should help anyone come a great deal closer to the ideal of a healthy mind in a healthy body.

CHAPTER 22

Raising Happier Children

If it is true, as this book has attempted to demonstrate, that a person's emotional patterns have a great deal to do with his ultimate susceptibility or resistance to cancer and other major diseases, then the best time to build emotional resistance to cancer would certainly be in childhood. In the adult, emotional patterns are well established and hard to alter. Their structure is held rigid by the mental process known as "rationalization." We can illustrate what rationalization means with some examples.

Let us say we are dealing with a recently widowed woman whose children are grown. She has lost the entire focus of her devotion and her reasons for living. Yet she puts up a brave front of cheerfulness, and seeing that her sorrow is deeply suppressed, we recognize that she has fallen into an emotional pattern related to the incidence of cancer. We might try to advise her that she would be better off to let her sorrow come to the surface and express it, but if we did, the chances are that she would have very good, rational arguments about why that would be a bad thing to do. She might say that she feels other people are a great deal worse off than she is, or that she has had more out of life than most, or that it isn't fair to go around inflicting your unhappiness on others. In other words, she has built up a structure of intellectual belief that makes her emotional pattern seem the only correct one to her. Consequently she will not change, is probably unable to change, and we are very afraid that she is becoming susceptible to a fatal disease.

The teenage girl who is afraid of boys may argue with conviction that boys are rough unpredictable animals rather than admit that there is anything irrational about her fears. The mother who overprotects her children can just about convince you that permitting children any exposure to the hazards of life is unforgivable neglect.

So there is not much hope that you can go to a mature man or woman who has spent an entire life of unwonted self-sacrifice and buried unhappiness and persuade that person to change before it is too late. As a matter of fact, a number of the research studies that have been reported in this book have shown that it was actually possible for someone skilled enough to predict the future occurrence of cancer in people not yet showing any diagnostic sign of the disease, on the basis of firmly established patterns of personality. If it had been possible to persuade such people to change their patterns, we can be sure that those studying them would have done so.

But every doctor knows that even though he is constantly advising his patients that they have to relax, have some fun, get away for a good rest, etc., either such advice is not followed, or even when it is, it rarely does any good. If a man has spent 50 years persuading himself that he must not relax, a few words are not going to change him.

Thus it would seem a far more fruitful approach to consider what we, as parents, can do to help our children establish healthful patterns of personality and avoid those patterns that in the long run might lead to serious disease. Scientists concerned with the relationship between emotions and disease have begun to investigate precisely this question. One very interesting study was made by two Philadelphia doctors, Claus Bahne Bahnson and Marjorie Brooks Bahnson of the Department of Psychiatry of Jefferson Medical College. They reported on their study to the Annual Meeting of the Eastern Psychological Association in Washington, D.C. in April, 1968. The Bahnsons used four groups of people for their study, the groups being matched as to age. Three of these groups comprised coronary heart disease, cancer and hemophilia patients while the fourth control group consisted of well, normal men. All four groups were given the same extensive thoroughly tested questionnaires and checked by personal interviews to determine what kind of relationships had existed with their parents and what their emotional reactions as children were.

In this study, of course, we are most interested in the cancer group and the normal controls, for if we can learn some principles of child raising that will help our children to grow up free of disease, we will have learned a great deal.

"With respect to maternal attitudes," say the Bahnsons, "cancer patients consistently rate their mothers lower than well controls on both positive and negative dimensions, e.g., protective and loving, or rejective and punitive. . . . Cancer patients remember their mothers as people who did not relate closely to them one way or the other, and who did not invest affectively in them. A perspective of coldness and barrenness in their perception of their mothers emerges from these ratings."

Although this result is not phrased in the language in which an individual would ordinarily put it, its meaning is perfectly clear. These cancer patients when they were children felt that their mothers did not really want them. This does not mean that the mothers failed to go through all the forms of duty fulfillment that are generally expected of parents. Children may have been fed on schedule and fed well. Their clothes may have been kept in good condition, they may have been sent to Sunday School and given the best education that money can buy. Their parents may have supervised their friendships, encouraged their talents, performed every "duty" of a parent. But if you have no emotional involvement with your children, if you are going through the forms more for what other people will think of you than for the child himself, somehow it is always impossible to hide that essential fact from the youngster. And if there is anything that the Bahnson study establishes, it is that there is no substitute for love in the relations between parents and child. Children can do without a great deal and never feel deprived in a warm and loving family. But all the luxuries money can buy are no substitute for that warmth and love.

It is interesting that among the group of cancer patients studied by the Bahnsons there was no particularly strong feeling of neglect by parents, any more than there was among the control group of well people. But while both groups felt that they got adequate care and attention from their parents, there was a much stronger feeling in the cancer group that somehow their mothers had rejected them and did not truly love them.

It is easy to see how such a conviction in a child will lead to an inability to give love that the child feels is always rejected, and in time create that deep sense of alienation that we have previously found to be an important part of the personalities of cancer victims.

The Bahnsons say that "Cancer patients also describe their fathers as non-protective and non-involved . . . The very low ratings on father's protectiveness by the cancer group achieved the highest significance of any one comparison with the well group in this study."

And this is most interesting for it indicates how enormously important to a child's entire future development is a strong father. Symbolically and actually, the father is the protector of the entire family. Children are small, weak and relatively helpless, and they know it. As they can rely on a father's protection, they are relatively strong and secure through the father's strength and security. But if through either weakness or lack of interest the father fails to fulfill his protective role, the children cannot help but feel an accentuated helplessness in a hostile world. Such a feeling of helplessness, we have seen, is another well-defined aspect of the cancer-prone personality.

"One gains the impression of a real vacuum in these patients' lives due to a lack of parental security and protectiveness," state the Bahnsons. "Cancer patients felt emotionally deprived during childhood and had insufficient emotional contact with their parents. . . . It is obvious that subjectively cancer patients are even more disappointed about their mothers than about their fathers, although both are seen in a negative light."

Much of the above we might have guessed. What will come as a surprise to many, is that in the Bahnson's study it turned out that the cancer patients had less demanded of them by their parents and were not punished as frequently or as severely as the healthy controls were by their parents.

This we consider an extremely important aspect of the problem of how to raise a child to produce a physically and emotionally healthy adult. Above all else, apparently, what the child needs is security. And security is a very different thing from indulgence. Parents who do not deeply love their children very often over-indulge them as a substitute or a pretense of love. But what the child needs is to have his own place in the world and to know exactly what that place is. He needs to have duties, he needs to know exactly what he may do and may not do, he needs to know that he is safe and protected as long as he behaves properly and that he will be punished if he oversteps the line.

To put the same matter in another way, parents should not be afraid of their own emotions. They should not try to raise their children too much by the book or by the dictates of their intellectual judgments. It is better to permit the exaggerated responses of punishment rather than reasoning when the child has aroused your fears, and of caresses rather than verbal approval when the child merits them. Both give the child better assurance of being loved and protected. Both will help the child to grow into a healthy adult with the kind of zest for life that makes it far more likely the onslaughts of disease will be resisted and overcome.

CHAPTER 23

Conclusion

AT THIS POINT, instead of writing a conclusion I should say, "Now start at the beginning and read it over again —then let me talk to you." But we can't wait, we must cap the book with some kind of conclusion right now, and here.

The theme is that happy people rarely get cancer, so the problem is to develop a spirit of happiness. I refer you to chapter 5 about those happy Italians at Roseto, Pennsylvania. Their happiness comes from their good health.

In chapter 3 we similarly showed that the Hunza people of Northern India are happy because they're healthy. Cancer is an unknown disease there. So problem number one is to get yourself into good health, by a healthful diet, and the taking of exercise, walking as much as possible. Getting your body into a healthy condition is a step away from cancer. So hitch your wagon to some good health program. You will find PREVENTION magazine a specific method for the attainment of optimum health.

Then develop positive thinking. Become more optimistic! It can be gradually cultivated. Your body physically changes every so many years—so can your character.

A book to read which you can get in the library is *Food and Character* by Louis Berman, M.D. On the jacket of this book appears the following:

"Glands grow more and more important as we come to know more about them. We know that human beings differ fundamentally in personality, character, physique, appearance, and general behavior because of differences in these little mysterious glands. What makes these differences?

"Dr. Berman takes up systematically the fundamental discoveries in food research from the earliest times until the present day. He considers the function of different food elements and the underlying pattern in the construction of a diet. The relation of these to the different ductless glands is then taken up in detail and the author shows how different food elements, including the vitamins and minerals, may change personality characteristics. Dr. Berman's thesis shows that special foods, by affecting the glands, may be used to change personality and make for a more favorable development of character."

A bright, happy disposition can be cultivated. You must work at it. Part of this problem is to develop a sense of humor if you don't already have one. Look for and encourage the humorous. Watch it on T.V., at the movies and the legitimate theatre. If necessary get joke books and read them once in awhile.

A happy disposition and a sense of humor can be life saving. It has been discovered in mining disasters, when 7 or 8 miners are trapped at the bottom of a shaft, if at least one of them is a lively, happy person with a good sense of humor, the group will live much longer.

In this respect I must relate a true story relative to an electric manufacturing company which I own—The Rodale Mfg. Co., Inc. of Emmaus, Penna. During the depression when money became very scarce we couldn't make the payments on our building mortgage. At that time I was editing a humorous magazine called *The American Humorist.*

One day I received a call to come to the bank at Emmaus which held our mortgage. I sensed the worst. The bank's attorney, Senator Snyder, was there. I was surprised to hear him make his little speech. He said, after a few preliminaries, "I happen to be a reader of Mr. Rodale's *American Humorist.* In my opinion such a happy man must be honest, and if we give him time he will work his way out of his difficulties."

The bank gave me time and we worked our way out of the tight squeeze we were in. Today the Rodale Mfg. Co. is a very large, profitable business, employing about 400 persons.

One of the ways to keep happy is to have a hobby or two. It should be begun now, not when a bereavement occurs, at which time the climate is not encouraging for the starting of hobbies. You can buy books devoted to hobbies, but I would like to suggest one that you might find interesting. Choose a subject that might be covered in your daily newspaper and paste clippings on the subject in a scrapbook. Examples of subjects can be animals, insects, individual countries like France, Germany, etc., the astronauts, colleges, juvenile delinquency, air pollution, the theatre, education methods, etc.

Just as I finished this paragraph we received a visit of my daughter-in-law, Ardath, Robert's wife, and their 5 children, our grandchildren. We sat around for awhile then suddenly I said, "Heather, Heidi and David," they were the 3 oldest, 13, 15 and 16, "I have a proposition," and I described the idea of keeping a scrapbook of newspaper clippings on one subject. "If you will choose a subject and get 100 pages of average scrapbook size filled with clippings on that subject, I will give each of you $50. I will pay $25 when you finish 50 pages and the balance on the completion of the 100 pages."

You should have seen the flurry of interest that created. Heather chose New Methods of Education, Heidi, Archaeology and David the Hippies. It was Sunday and the *N.Y. Times, The Allentown Call,* and *The Philadelphia Inquirer* lay strewn about our living room. They began to tear into them. I also permitted *Time* and *Newsweek* and any other newspaper to be used.

I impressed upon them the sense of creation and achievement involved and I told them they must read each item and think about it, but that they need not write anything about it. I realized that I had done a wonderful thing, because this activity would work upon them and influence their way of thinking and working in the future, including the development of the ability to concentrate, thus improving their school work. It just goes to show you, it pays to write books, because you get ideas as you go along. Oh yes, one of the rules of the clipping game was that I had to approve the subjects they chose.

Now coming back to our conclusion and the subject of hobbies.

Years ago I was invited to talk about organic gardening to a botany class at Wellesley College of which my daughter Ruth was a member; as editor of *Organic Gardening and Farming* magazine I am supposed to be a sort of authority on the subject. I was told that a 93-year-old man, who lived nearby, would be in the audience because of the wonderful experience he had had with the organic method in his garden. This method consists of the avoidance of the use of commercial fertilizers and poisonous insecticides, substituting composts made from animal manure, weeds, leaves, etc.

It seems that this man's wife had died a few years back and the shock and grief had taken from him his will to live. This man had been a gardener all his life. A friend told him about organic gardening. The idea appealed to him, and he began to apply it in his garden with great zeal and success. When he heard that I was to talk to the botany class he asked to be permitted to come so that he could thank me in person.

This man had substituted something for his grief. He did not have to sit around and think of his helpmate. Even during the winter he was planning his program for the next spring. He had added years to his life.

Everyone should have a full life. The mind should be made happy with activity. Thus the habit of happiness will be assured.

Now I would like to make an important observation with regard to our problem, and that is the use of hypnosis when a shock occurs to an older person. Many people have wrong ideas on the subject. They visualize the stage hypnotist's dog tricks with his victims. In actual practice today hypnosis is gaining wide recognition and acceptance as a method of improving one's health and getting rid of obnoxious habits. The hypnotist does not put you to sleep. You are awake, but in a half drowsed state. You can hear him talking to you and to your subconscious mind. He speaks to you as a soothing source of inspiration, guides your mind to accept trouble in a philosophical sort of way. He sort of preaches a sermon to you. He might speak thus: "Your dear wife has passed away, but she wouldn't want you to grieve yourself to death because of it. Remember she will always be a pleasant memory to you, but she will not want you to stop living, etc., etc., etc."

Hypnosis is accepted by the medical profession and the psychiatrists, for it has produced excellent results. You will find names of hypnotists in the yellow pages of your telephone book.

Is hatred a factor in shortening one's life and causing cancer? The act of hating affects one's breathing, it reduces the oxygenation of the body's tissues and depresses the respiration of the cells. It's a known fact that anger, anxiety and resentment can weaken capillary walls. I am leading up to such things as the hatred of anti-semitism and the hatred of the Negro's racist activities, and even the hatred of one's mother-in-law. How about the hatred "enjoyed" by the Russian communists? Could Stalin have lived longer had he not hated with such venom? Will the present day demonstrating and violent activities of students and Negroes give them more cancer?

A young Negro fellow about 25 passed in front of me on Madison Avenue in New York City, a few weeks ago, his face distorted with hate. He said, "Man, you're on my land," and kept on moving. What kind of life is that with this hate always uppermost in this fellow's mind?

If you follow the cancer statistics you will find that this dread disease is getting more prevalent year by year. Harry Golden said a year ago, "In recent weeks there seems to be a more intense hatred. Even in the '50's there was some attempt to argue, but now there's no argument, just plain unadulterated hatred." There is no question about it—the tensions are increasing, and we may expect this to further increase the incidence of cancer.

Index

A

Alcohol . . . . p. 188

B

Bahnson, Claus Bahne and Marjorie Brooks . . . . pp. 69, 197
Baltrusch, Dr. Hans-Joachim F. . . . . . . p. 80
Blood sugar,
and cancer . . . . pp. 54-58
and emotional change . . . . pp. 48-58
Bone meal . . . . p. 193
Booth, Dr. Gotthard . . . . p. 83
Bread . . . . p. 189

C

Cancer-prone personality . . . . pp. 68-76, 108-110, 124-128, 130-135
Case histories . . . . pp. 95-99, 106-108, 110-120, 142-147, 160-163
Cheraskin, Dr. E. . . . . p. 54
Children, emotional change . . . . pp. 130-136, 139-141, 195-201
Coffee and tea . . . . p. 189
Creative work . . . . pp. 93-95

D

Drugs, for mental depression . . . . pp. 60-61

E

Eggs . . . . p. 189
Emotional damage, in childhood . . . . pp. 130-136
Emotional shock, and cancer . . . . pp. 122-123
Emotions, as cancer causers . . . . pp. 42-47

Euphoria .... pp. 178-181
Evans, Dr. Elida .... p. 89
Extraverted personality .... pp. 92-93, 104-106, 109

G

Gardening-cancer hypothesis .... pp. 8-12
Glands, and emotional stress .... pp. 149-151
Greene, Dr. William A., Jr. .... pp. 158, 165

H

Happiness-cancer relationship .... pp. 3-5
Heart disease statistics .... pp. 29-32
Hill walking .... pp. 32-34, 182-186
Hodgkin's disease .... pp. 137-147
Hormones, and cancer .... pp. 150-151
Hunzas .... pp. 13-20, 23-25
Hypoglycemia .... p. 49

I

Intelligence .... p. 142
Isolation, and Hodgkin's disease ..... pp. 137-147

K

Kissen, Dr. David M. .... pp. 42, 152

L

Leigh, Dr. Denis .... p. 44
LeShan, Lawrence, Ph.D. .... pp. 77, 126, 129, 138
Leukemia, and emotions .... pp. 158-169
Lung cancer, smoking and emotions .. pp. 42-44, 152-156

M

McCarrison, Sir Robert .... pp. 13, 15
Marriage, and hypoglycemia .... p. 50
Masor, Dr. Nathan .... p. 61

INDEX

Meat .... p. 189
Mice, an organic experiment .... pp. 45-47
Milk .... p. 190
Ministers, and cancer patients .... pp. 83-88

N

Nagyri .... pp. 21-28
Negroes, cancer statistics .... pp. 6-7
Nix, J. T., Ph.D. .... p. 170
Nuns .... pp. 170-176
Nutrition,
of the Hunzans .... pp. 17-20
and personality change .... pp. 49-58
the Rosetan diet .... pp. 36-39

O

Object loss .... pp. 159-160
Ogilvie, Sir Heneage .... pp. 1-7
Oppenheimer, Dr. J. Robert .... p. 79
Organic farming .... pp. 34-35
Organically raised food .... p. 190

P

Parents, and children's emotions ..... pp. 198-201
Personality, cancer-prone .... pp. 68-76, 108-110, 124-128, 130-135
PREVENTION Program for Health .. pp. 187-194
Protein .... p. 190
Psychosomatic causes of cancer ...... pp. 89-120
Psychosomatic research .... pp. 80-82

Q

Questionnaire, cancer-prone
personality .... pp. 71-72

R

Rakoff, Dr. A. E. .... p. 148

Religion, ministers and cancer .... pp. 83-88
Roberts, Dr. Sam .... pp. 49, 52-53
Rosenfeld, Dr. Cecelia .... p. 50
Roseto, Pennsylvania .... pp. 29-41
Ruby, Jack .... pp. 44-45

S

Salt .... p. 190
Seeds .... p. 190
Sheridan, Ann .... p. 45
Sleep .... p. 191
Soil, electricity and magnetism ...... pp. 10-11
Sugar .... pp. 39-41, 191
Suicide, and cancer .... pp. 77-82

T

Temperament, and cancer .... p. 121
Thyroid gland, and mental health .... pp. 61-67
Tobacco .... p. 191

U

Unsaturated fatty acids .... p. 191

V

Vitamin and mineral supplements .... p. 192

W

Walking .... pp. 177-186, 193
Water-softeners .... p. 194
Women, emotions and leukemia ..... pp. 165-169

Y

Yudkin, Dr. John .... p. 39